FOOD ALLERGIES

FOOD ALLERGIES

Alice C. Richer

Biographies of Disease
Julie K. Silver, M.D., Series Editor

GREENWOOD PRESS
Westport, Connecticut • London

Library of Congress Cataloging-in-Publication Data

Richer, Alice C.
  Food allergies / Alice C. Richer.
    p. ; cm. — (Biographies of disease, ISSN 1940-445X)
  Includes bibliographical references and index.
  ISBN 978-0-313-35273-7 (alk. paper)
  1. Food allergy. I. Title. II. Series: Biographies of disease.
[DNLM: 1. Food Hypersensitivity. 2. Risk Factors. WD 310 R529f 2009]
  RC596.R53 2009
  616.97′5—dc22   2008052246

British Library Cataloguing in Publication Data is available.

Library of Congress Catalog Card Number: 2008052246
ISBN: 978-0-313-35273-7
ISSN: 1940-445X

First published in 2009

Greenwood Press, 88 Post Road West, Westport, CT 06881
An imprint of Greenwood Publishing Group, Inc.
www.greenwood.com

Printed in the United States of America

∞™

The paper used in this book complies with the
Permanent Paper Standard issued by the National
Information Standards Organization (Z39.48–1984).

10 9 8 7 6 5 4 3 2 1

This book is dedicated to my sister Rose, who lives with a debilitating gastrointestinal disorder and food intolerance.

"Give thanks to the Lord, for he is good...." *Psalm 136*

Contents

Tables and Figures

TABLES

FIGURES

Series Foreword

E very disease has a story to tell: about how it started long ago and began to disable or even take the lives of its innocent victims, about the way it hurts us, and about how we are trying to stop it. In this Biographies of Disease series, the authors tell the stories of the diseases that we have come to know and dread.

The stories of these diseases have all of the components that make for great literature. There is incredible drama played out in real-life scenes from the past, present, and future. You'll read about how men and women of science stumbled trying to save the lives of those they aimed to protect. Turn the pages and you'll also learn about the amazing success of those who fought for health and won, often saving thousands of lives in the process.

If you don't want to be a health professional or research scientist now, when you finish this book you may think differently. The men and women in this book are heroes who often risked their own lives to save or improve ours. This is the biography of a disease, but it is also the story of real people who made incredible sacrifices to stop it in its tracks.

Julie K. Silver, M.D.
Assistant Professor, Harvard Medical School
Department of Physical Medicine and Rehabilitation

Preface

Food allergies are a growing concern worldwide. Hospital admissions for food allergies in the United Kingdom increased by 500 percent since 1990, and an estimated twelve million Americans report living with a food allergy. Almost seven million of them are allergic to seafood and three million to peanuts or tree nuts. Two million school-age children in the United States are diagnosed with food allergies, and pediatric peanut allergies doubled from 1997 to 2002. This trend is mirrored in other developed and industrialized nations as well. Concerns prompted the European Union in 2005 to begin a multidisciplinary project, known as EuroPrevall, to study the problem and develop diagnostic tools and databases. The "Exploratory Investigations in Food Allergy" program in the United States was launched in 2008 to investigate the origin, epidemiology, and genetics of food allergy as well as encourage new investigators to enter this growing research area.

While treatment for many environmental allergens allows effective control of them, this is not the case with food allergies. Food is an integral part of life. Avoidance of a food allergen is critical, but often very difficult to do. Eliminating one or more food groups can cause poor growth or health, chronic diseases, and eating disorders. Enjoyment of social activities, frequently centered on food, may decrease and lead to depression and isolation. Although food allergies and hypersensitivities are a serious threat to life, it is a reality that is not always respected or understood by those who take food for granted.

This book will prove to be a valuable resource for students, consumers, health care professionals, and anyone who cares for or lives with a food allergy or hypersensitivity. Chapter 1 discusses food allergy incidence worldwide, the science of immunology, and how the immune system works. The differences between a food allergy, a food intolerance or hypersensitivity, and food-related medical disorders are differentiated. Chapter 2 describes symptoms of adverse food reactions and current diagnostic methods. Questionable testing methods offered to a vulnerable public are also explored. Chapter 3 delves into theories and possible causes for food allergies. Clinical studies are looked at and guidelines for use when evaluating research study relevance are provided. A select list of some of the more important clinical studies is also presented.

Chapter 4 outlines how to live in the real world with a food allergy or hypersensitivity. Food-labeling laws and ingredient terminology are reviewed. Each food allergy is analyzed, associated terms for each of them are listed, and a comprehensive listing of allergenic or problematic foods and ingredients are provided. Cross-contamination risks, an ever-present danger, are discussed as well. Chapter 5 educates the reader about how to respond during a severe food allergy reaction and reviews treatment steps that should be taken. Signs and symptoms that indicate an anaphylactic reaction is imminent are reviewed. Chapter 6 discusses the psychological effects food allergies can have and ways to cope with these at home, when grocery shopping, or when eating away from home. Challenges that face teenagers and young adults, who are at the highest risk for fatal anaphylactic reactions, are examined. Chapter 7 reviews new research areas and possible diagnostic methods and future treatments on the horizon.

A Question and Answer section addresses uncommon situations that may be encountered. The Appendices provide a listing of non-allergenic foods that provide the many important nutrients found in allergenic foods as well as a resource listing of government Web sites, organizations, and food companies that will improve the management of food allergies in the real world. *Food Allergies* should prove to be a valuable resource for everyone.

Acknowledgments

M any thanks to Cathy Weiner for her loyal friendship and editing prowess and to Julie Silver who is a true inspiration. I am grateful for Julie's confidence and support, which made this book a reality. Thank you for allowing me to be a part of this important education series.

Introduction

A nxiety. Fear. Frustration. Panic. These are just some of the emotions people and their families struggle with when they live with a food allergy. The human immune system, responsible for protecting us from harmful and deadly microorganisms, malfunctions and comes to perceive food as a threatening substance. For reasons still not clearly understood, this abnormal immune response to a substance that is so essential for survival triggers adverse reactions that range from mild to life threatening. The result often leads to poor nutritional intake affecting health (and growth in children), eating disorders, depression, and sometimes death.

Most people assume they have a food allergy after suffering an adverse reaction to a food, yet only a very small percentage of these reactions are classified as "true" food allergies. Approximately 1–2 percent of adults and 5–7 percent of children in developed countries live with a diagnosed food allergy. However, food allergy incidence appears to be on the increase worldwide. Peanut allergies doubled in children from 1997 to 2002 in the United States. Asthma, a reliable indicator of food allergy susceptibility, increased 100 percent over the past thirty years (although other factors may have contributed). Food allergy reactions increased hospital admissions by 500 percent in the United Kingdom since 1990.

More than 200 foods are reported to cause adverse reactions. However, in reality, only eight foods—eggs, fish, milk, peanuts, shellfish, soy, tree nuts (almonds, cashews, pecans, pistachios, walnuts), and wheat—are actually responsible for more than 90 percent of diagnosed food allergy reactions worldwide. Concerns about food allergy increases prompted the European Union to initiate EuroPrevall in 2005, a multidisciplinary project involving more than twenty countries, to study food allergies and develop diagnostic tools and databases. In August 2008 in the United States, the National Institutes of Health (NIH), the National Institute of Allergy and Infectious Diseases (NIAID), the Environmental Protection Agency (EPA), and some nonprofit food allergy organizations committed research funds for a new food allergy research program called "Exploratory Investigations in Food Allergy." The focus of this program is on investigating the origin, epidemiology, and genetics of food allergy as well as to encourage new investigators to enter this growing research area.

However, food allergy reactions are not the only adverse food reactions causing concern. Other food hypersensitivities and medical conditions can mimic symptoms similar to those of a food allergy. Inborn metabolic disorders, food-related medical disorders, and adverse reactions to food additives are also capable of producing symptoms that can become life-threatening. Correctly diagnosing the cause of an adverse food reaction is challenging, because many other diseases or environmental chemicals can cause similar symptoms. Added to this is the problem of "hidden food allergens." Many processed foods or restaurant meals may contain unsuspected food allergens. Food allergens can "go" airborne and trigger a severe reaction in susceptible people. Food allergens can "lurk" on the surface of food-processing equipment, restaurant tables, or school desks. School bullying, currently on the increase, may involve intentional contamination of an allergic schoolmate's lunch with a food allergen, putting that child's life in danger. The "real world" can be a very dangerous place when living with a food allergy or hypersensitivity. Many of those who live with them wonder if it is even possible to exist and live a "normal" life.

The good news is it is possible to enjoy foods, remain healthy, and live a life free of fear. The tools to accomplish this are provided in this book. Food allergies and hypersensitivities are a serious threat to life, a reality that is not always understood by those who take eating for granted. This book educates the reader about the human immune system and why adverse food reactions occur. Differences between a "true" food allergy and other food-related conditions that can trigger adverse symptoms and diagnostic methods used are discussed. What to do in an emergency and advice about preventing adverse reactions are detailed. Immunology science and food allergy research are explored. New research areas and future treatments and diagnostic methods on the horizon are examined. Food regulations are reviewed and tips and strategies to use in the home, supermarket, restaurant, or anywhere outside of the home are outlined. Comprehensive listings of allergenic or problematic foods and ingredients are provided. Finally, resources that can assist individuals and their families to cope with the realities of the world of food are documented.

Food Allergies will prove to be a valuable resource for students, consumers, health care professionals, and anyone who cares for or lives with a food allergy.

1

When Foods Turn Deadly

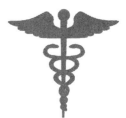

"What is food to one is bitter poison to another."

—Lucretius

Food plays a significant and important role in our lives, both for good health as well as social well-being. Religious holidays, family celebrations, and social gatherings often include special dishes made just for the occasion. Then there are birthdays, sporting events, ice cream socials, movies, weddings, ad infinitum, where food is included as an integral part of the event. But for those living with a food allergy, special occasions or a visit to a friend's house can turn into a deadly experience.

Take the case of Grant Freeman, a thirty-eight-year-old businessman from Australia. Mr. Freeman, who experienced adverse reactions after eating peanuts, tree nuts, eggs, seafood, and chicken, assumed he was allergic to these foods. Although he had never experienced any severe reactions prior to this event, he was always very careful to read food labels and ask how a meal was prepared before eating it. In April 2007 Mr. Freeman attended a business dinner at a local restaurant. Little did he suspect it would literally be his last supper. The restaurant Mr. Freeman dined at had been notified about his "food allergies" and took extra care to prepare a meal that would be "safe" for him to eat. According to a colleague who also attended the dinner, Mr. Freeman took a sip of wine and one bite of his tomato-based meal, declared something was wrong and that he didn't feel good, and collapsed. Unfortunately, he did not have an EpiPen with him—a device that administers medication that could have saved his life. Mr. Freeman lapsed into a coma after suffering severe brain damage. He was removed from life support two days later (Johnston, April 2007, *New Zealand Herald*). Could this terrible tragedy have been prevented? The answer is an emphatic yes.

While it would be nice to eat anything and everything without a care in the world, it is just not realistic for anyone who experiences a food allergy or hypersensitivity. For reasons still not fully understood, the human immune system reacts abnormally to some foods. So is it even possible to eat safely, enjoy social gatherings, and stay healthy when living with adverse food reactions? No matter what food a person struggles with, there is a way to stay "safe," consume all the nutrients necessary for good health, and still enjoy life. This chapter explores the science of immunology, the human immune system, and how and why adverse food reactions occur.

ARE FOOD ALLERGIES ON THE RISE?

The Centers for Disease Control and Prevention (CDC) estimates approximately twelve million Americans (three million of whom are children) experience some type of adverse reaction to a food. An estimated 30,000 Americans are rushed to emergency rooms for severe food reactions and between 100 and 200 die from food-related anaphylaxis annually (CDC, September 2007, http://www.cdc.gov). Food allergies are not, however, restricted to just the United States. In Europe and most developed countries, an estimated 1–2 percent of adults and 5–7 percent of children have reported food allergies, making them a worldwide concern.

More than 200 foods are reported to cause adverse reactions, and most people assume they are allergic to a food after experiencing an adverse reaction. However, in reality, only eight foods—eggs, fish, milk, peanuts, shellfish, soy, tree nuts (almonds, cashews, pecans, pistachios, walnuts), and wheat—are actually responsible for over 90 percent of true food allergy reactions worldwide (Food Allergy & Anaphylaxis Network, http://www.foodallergy.org). Other medical conditions or food hypersensitivities can mimic symptoms similar to those of a food allergy. Prevalence of adverse food reactions varies regionally and is largely influenced by a country's dietary habits and food preparation methods. In the United States, eggs, milk, and peanut allergies are the most prevalent food allergies affecting children. Fish, peanuts, tree nuts, and

Table 1.1
Food Allergies around the World

Country	Allergy Prevalence	Common Food Allergens
Australia	1 to 2 percent of population	Eggs Fish Milk Peanut Sesame Shellfish Soy Tree nuts
Canada	1 to 2 percent of population; 2 to 8 percent among children	Eggs Fish Milk Peanut Sesame seeds Shellfish Sulfite additives Soy Tree nuts Wheat
Germany	2 to 3 percent of population; 3 to 6 percent among children; 30 percent in high risk groups (i.e., asthma)	Children: Eggs Fish Milk Peanuts Soy Tree nuts Wheat Adults: Eggs Fish Milk Peanut Shellfish Soy Pip/stone fruits (i.e., apple, peach) Tree nuts Vegetables (celery, carrot) Wheat
Italy	6 to 8 percent of population	Cow's milk Fish

(*continued*)

Table 1.1 (*continued*)

Country	Allergy Prevalence	Common Food Allergens
		Hen's Eggs
		Peanut
		Tree nuts
		Wheat
The Netherlands	Approximately 800,000 people	Eggs
		Fish
		Milk
		Peanut
		Sesame seed
		Shellfish
		Soy
		Tree nuts
		Wheat
New Zealand	Unknown	Eggs
		Fish
		Milk
		Peanut
		Shellfish
		Soy
		Tree nuts
		Wheat
United Kingdom	1 to 2 percent of the adult population; 5 to 8 percent in children under 16 years of age	Eggs
		Fish
		Milk
		Peanut
		Sesame seeds
		Shellfish
		Tree nuts
United States	12 million Americans	Eggs
		Fish
		Milk
		Peanut
		Shellfish
		Soy
		Tree nuts
		Wheat

Sources: Food Allergy & Anaphylaxis Alliance, "Food Allergy Around the World" (September 2008), http://www.foodallergyalliance.org/foo.html and EuroPrevall, "EuroPrevall: The Prevalence, Cost and Basis of Food Allergy across Europe" (September 2008), http://www.functionalfoodnet.eu.

shellfish commonly affect American adults. In Australia, Denmark, and Sweden, cow's milk allergy is quite common in infants and children under the age of two. In Southeast Asian countries, such as Japan and South Korea, buckwheat allergies are prevalent. In China, where peanut consumption (in the form of boiled or fried peanuts) is the same as in the United States (in the form of dry roasted peanuts, which makes the protein allergens stronger), peanut allergies are negligible. In Israel, where peanuts are also a staple of the daily diet, sesame seed allergies are far more common than peanut allergies.

Many experts believe food allergies associated with life-threatening anaphylaxis are on the rise worldwide. Although studies have yet to prove this beyond a shadow of a doubt, some data does suggest that they are on the increase. Pediatric peanut allergies doubled from 1997 to 2002 in the United States. Since 1990, food allergy reactions increased hospital admissions by 500 percent in the United Kingdom. Asthma cases, a reliable predictor of food allergy susceptibility, increased 100 percent over the past thirty years (although other factors, such as air pollution, may play a role) (Wood, 2007). Increasing global travel and the importation of food products from other countries also expose populations to new foods. For example, in the United States kiwi allergies were uncommon until recently as this fruit (indigenous to China) becomes increasingly popular in America. Increasing concerns about food hypersensitivities prompted the European Union in 2005 to begin a multidisciplinary project, known as EuroPrevall, to study the problem and develop diagnostic tools and databases.

While theories abound, there are still no clear-cut reasons for these increases. Family genetics appear to play a key role in food allergy susceptibility. Research studies performed with twins found that when one twin has a peanut allergy, an identical twin will have a 64 percent chance of having a peanut allergy as well. However, a non-identical twin only has a 7 percent chance of sharing the same peanut allergy (Wood, 2007). Although this confirms a strong genetic link to food allergy susceptibility, experts in the field believe a combination of genetics and environmental factors are the cause of many food allergies and hypersensitivities. Certainly, increased awareness about food allergies today has led to improved detection and diagnosis, yet better detection doesn't totally account for the dramatic increases being seen. Some theories point to ingredients and food additives used in commercially prepared foods, increased use of vitamin supplements and antacids, exposure to tobacco smoke, living in a "too clean" environment with lack of exposure to germs that build up immunity, introducing food at too young an age, and use of bioengineered foods as culprits. Much more research still needs to be done.

When U. S. scientists first began to bioengineer food, the first food they selected to modify was the soy plant, a relatively inexpensive source of protein. Scientists wanted to develop a disease-resistant plant that would increase the yield of soy nuts. To do this, they took genetic material from Brazil nuts and inserted it into soy plants. However, the Brazil nut is a tree nut and one of a group of nuts that often trigger severe allergic reactions. Thus, the potential for widespread life-threatening allergic reactions was astronomical. Fortunately, scientists realized the potential hazard and removed this plant from production. Industry safeguards against a similar modification in the future were implemented, and bioengineered foods must now be labeled. But this one example highlights the potential danger to consumers when foods are modified from their natural state and the need for consumers to be vigilant about what they eat.

IMMUNOLOGY—THE SCIENCE

We now know adverse food allergies are caused by an abnormal immune response. Immunology is the science that studies the human immune system. One deadly plague that highlights the history of immunological science is small-pox. Smallpox, an infectious virus responsible for an estimated 300–500 million deaths in just the twenthieth century alone, was a common and deadly plague worldwide for many centuries. Evidence of smallpox lesions has been found on the remains of Egyptian mummies, and numerous historical texts record smallpox plagues. Historians believe smallpox first appeared around 10,000 BC in Africa, spreading worldwide as trade increased and discoveries were made in the New World (Reidel, 2005). As far back as 5,000 BC, a connection was noted between surviving an illness and immunity. The Greek historian Thucydides recorded the devastation to the Greek population during the Athenian Plague (430–426 BC). Of particular interest is the fact that he also noted that those who survived became immune to it and were then employed to take care of the sick.

Because smallpox was so deadly, various methods were tried to prevent infection. The French philosopher Voltaire reports that during the fifteenth century the Chinese and Turkish civilizations inhaled (like snuff) crushed up scabs from mild cases of smallpox (an early form of immunization). Inoculations (also called variolation because it was used specifically against smallpox) were used in Africa, China, and India before the eighteenth century. Inoculation, the method of introducing viruses to stimulate the immune system to develop protection against it, used a sharp instrument dipped in the pus of a lesion (such as a smallpox lesion) to push (inoculate) the pus (vaccine) under the skin in an uninfected person. This, in turn, stimulated the body to build a natural protection (immunity) against the disease while decreasing the risk of succumbing to it. Inoculations could also be given orally, by scraping the vaccine into the skin, or by injecting it into a muscle. This method did successfully protect some from smallpox, but it also put them at risk for developing a severe case of smallpox or contracting another bloodborne disease, such as syphilis, because the infected material contained live, infectious microorganisms.

During the eighteenth century, Lady Mary Wortley Montague introduced variolation in England. Having survived smallpox herself and losing her brother to the disease, she became a strong advocate of the practice and had her own children inoculated. In 1721, when the smallpox epidemic in Boston, Massachusetts, claimed half of the city's 12,000 inhabitants, Reverend Cotton Mather and Dr. Zabdiel Boylston successfully used variolation to reduce the death rate from 14 percent to 2 percent. But it wasn't until the late 1700s and 1800s, when medical science was in its infancy and many lifesaving discoveries were being made, that the science of immunology was born and vaccines with long-lasting immunization against deadly diseases were pioneered.

The English physician, Edward Jenner (1749–1822), conducted the first immunology experiment in 1796 and is credited as both the founder of immunology and with introducing vaccination to the world. The word "vaccine" originates from the word *Vacca*, which means "cow." It was common knowledge at the time that milkmaids who became ill with cowpox rarely came down with smallpox. The cowpox (vaccinia) virus is very similar in chemical structure to the smallpox (variola) virus. Thus, when ill with cowpox, the immune system makes antibodies that protect against future exposures to both cowpox and smallpox. Dr. Jenner theorized he could protect individuals from smallpox infection by inoculating them with the cowpox virus. With this knowledge in mind and hoping to protect an eight-year-old boy from smallpox, he injected the boy with pus from a cowpox boil. The boy developed a few mild symptoms, but no skin lesions. When his symptoms subsided, Dr. Jenner then injected him with smallpox. The boy was successfully immunized against smallpox and remained healthy. In 1798 Dr. Jenner published his findings and called the procedure "vaccination." Vaccination represented the first reliable method for granting immunity against contagious diseases, and vaccination methods today use weakened, dead, or purified viruses, toxins, or bacteria. Over time vaccinations replaced inoculations, and smallpox was declared eradicated worldwide in 1977. Although Dr. Jenner was one of the first in the scientific community to study and experiment with inoculations and vaccinations, his theories were controversial during his lifetime.

Not until Louis Pasteur (1822–1895), the French chemist who discovered that germs actually caused many infectious diseases, did the scientific and medical communities finally accept Dr. Jenner's work. Pasteur, considered by many to be the father of immunology and microbiology, made many important contributions to medicine. In the field of immunology, he is most famous for using attenuated (weakened) live viruses and bacteria as vaccines. Some of his more notable experiments immunized sheep and cattle against anthrax and saved a nine-year-old boy from rabies.

Robert Koch (1843–1910) continued Jenner's and Pasteur's work, winning a Nobel Prize in 1905 for his work in tuberculosis research. Elie Metchnikoff (1845–1916), Paul Ehrlich (1854–1915), Emil Adolph von Behring (1854–1917), Karl Landsteiner (1868–1943), and Charles Robert Richet (1850–1935) are only some of the more prominent physicians and scientists who advanced the study of immunology and discovered that the human immune system was far more complex than first realized. However, it wasn't until Carl Prausnitz-Giles (1876–1963), a German bacteriologist and immunologist who carried out extensive research on allergies and experimented specifically with food allergies, that food allergies were connected to the human immune system. The research team of Kimishige Ishizaka (1925–) and Terako Ishizaka also made the significant discovery of IgE, the immunoglobin intimately tied to food allergy reactions, as the principal agent of allergic reactions.

THE HUMAN IMMUNE SYSTEM

To understand why food allergies occur, it is necessary to be familiar with how the immune system works. Twelve systems are responsible for different functions of life—circulatory, digestive (gastrointestinal), endocrine, immune, lymphatic, muscular, nervous, reproductive, respiratory, skeletal, skin, and urinary. It is the immune system that is responsible for protecting humans from a daily assault of potentially life-threatening germs, viruses, pathogens, and chemicals. While some researchers think food allergies are due to a weak immune system, it is actually a strong immune system that becomes too protective and begins to identify some food components as threatening invaders that lead to adverse food reactions.

White blood cells, also called leukocytes, are responsible for immunity and are manufactured in many different areas of the body, circulating throughout the bloodstream and between organs. There are two primary types of leukocytes involved in allergic reactions: phagocytes and lymphocytes. Phagocytes destroy microorganisms that threaten health, and lymphocytes recognize foreign substances and assist in destroying them. Eosinophils, another type of leukocyte, sometimes become involved in the immune response as well. Two different types of lymphocytes become involved in the allergic response: B cells and T cells. B cells are formed and mature in the bone marrow. They are responsible for identifying invaders and defending against them. T cells are formed and mature in the thymus gland. They control the immune system and destroy invaders after they are identified.

So what triggers the immune system to go on "alert and go to battle"? When a foreign substance comes into the body, either through a cut, the air breathed, or via food or liquids consumed, the body immediately reacts. Most life-threatening intruders are bacteria, pathogens, viruses, or the toxins they produce. These invaders contain a component that the immune system identifies as threatening. This threatening component is called an antigen. Antigens are usually a protein, but can be a glycoprotein or a molecule linked to a protein. Antigens that trigger allergic reactions are known as allergens, and all allergens are antigens (although not all antigens are allergens).

When the body identifies a substance as an allergen, lymphocytes respond by releasing an antibody. An antibody is a protein that attaches itself to the intruder (allergen) so that the lymphocytes can distinguish between the "bad guy" and healthy tissue or normally safe substances (like foods). In response, two types of B cells are activated: mast cells and basophils. Mast cells are found in the respiratory tract, intestine, skin, and other body organs and are always "ready for action." Basophils "patrol" the bloodstream, alert for the "enemy." Both mast cells and basophils are armed at all times with special chemicals called inflammatory mediators (bradykinins, histamine, leukotrienes, or prostaglandins) that fight inflammation and destroy potentially harmful allergens.

Table 1.2
Function of Immunoglobulin Antibodies

Immunoglobulin Antibodies	Function
IgG	Primary circulating antibody. Attacks bacteria, pathogens, and viruses circulating in the bloodstream.
IgA	Found in breast milk, saliva, tears, and mucus. Attacks bacteria, pathogens, and viruses in the GI tract or breathing passages.
IgE	Rare antibody and a specialty cell that the immune system uses to fight parasitic infections. Involved in food allergy reactions.
IgD	A rare antibody and surface receptor on lymphocytes. Scientists remain uncertain of its function.
IgM	First antibody produced when an allergen is found or in response to immunizations. Traveling in clusters, they are very efficient at trapping viral infections and binding antigens together.

Five different types of antibodies, called immunoglobulin antibodies (Ig), are produced by lymphocytes. These immunoglobulin antibodies are IgA, IgD, IgE, IgG, and IgM, and each has a different responsibility. IgA, IgG, and IgM are the main antibodies that fight microorganisms and help to keep humans healthy and alive. IgE, mainly used to fight parasites, is the antibody that typically triggers allergic reactions. IgE is produced during the very first exposure to an allergen, which sensitizes the individual to that specific allergen. Thousands of IgE antibodies will then sit on the surface of mast cells and basophils. When exposed to this same allergen again, the IgE antibodies will recognize it and attach themselves to the allergen while also alerting the B cells. The B cells then "see" the allergen and begin to spray their chemicals directly at the allergen, destroying it before harm can be done. These types of allergic reactions are called IgE-mediated reactions.

T cell lymphocytes, along with dendritic cells (immune cells that activate T cells and are found on the skin and in the intestine, lungs, nose, and stomach) and intestinal epithelial cells, are also involved at the cellular level with

Table 1.3
Inflammatory Mediators

Chemical	Physical Response
Histamine	Blood vessel dilation
	Fluid and protein leakage via blood vessels, causing edema
	Mucus secretion increases
	Muscle contractions
	Stimulation of nerves, creating an "itch"
Bradykinins	Blood vessel dilation
Leukotrienes	Bronchospasms
Prostaglandins	Movement of cells containing inflammatory mediators
	Mucus secretion increases
	Muscle contractions, pain and swelling control responses
	Nervous system and gastrointestinal tract response
Th2 Cytokines:	Aching muscles
Interleukin 4 (IL-4)	Fatigue
Interleukin 5 (IL-5)	Fever
Interleukin 6 (IL-6)	Inflammation
Interleukin 13 (IL-13)	Itching
	Malaise
	Swelling

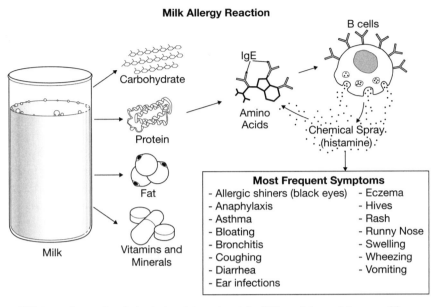

Milk Allergy Reaction

Milk is made up of carbohydrates, fat, and protein. Milk protein contains over 20 different amino acids. In an allergic reaction to milk, *IgE* attaches itself to an amino acid it finds threatening. Mast cells identify the allergen and spray the amino acid with chemicals to neutralize and destroy it. The chemical release causes allergy symptoms to develop.

Figure 1.1. Milk Allergy Reaction [Jeff Dixon].

intestinal immunity. When T cells are first activated, they respond by either alerting B cells to make IgE antibodies, alert other immune cells called eosinophils to respond, or activate both systems. When eosinophils are alerted, they travel to the area of alert and release chemicals called cytokines, which can cause an allergic reaction. T cell responses are either Th1 or Th2 responses; the type determines which cytokine chemicals are released. In the Th1 response, IgG or IgM antibodies are produced, *not* IgE, and disease-causing microorganisms are their usual target. In the Th2 response, IgE antibodies are produced and sometimes target nonthreatening substances like food. The Th2 cytokines can also influence mast cells to release inflammatory mediators. Delayed allergic reactions (allergic reactions can be either immediate or delayed) are influenced by the Th2 response. When T cells respond instead of B cells, these reactions are called cell-mediated reactions. Whether B cell or T cell produced, the effect of inflammatory mediators or cytokine chemicals on body tissues trigger allergy symptoms that can range from mild to severe.

So what does all this have to do with food allergies? Recall that IgE antibodies identify potentially threatening proteins in allergens like pollens, mold spores, bee venom, dust mites, and animal dander. All foods contain antigens, and some have proteins (made up of amino acid chains) along with other important nutrients. For example, milk has vitamins, minerals, carbohydrates, fat, and protein. All proteins are made up of a chain of amino acids. There are more than twenty different amino acids, and each amino acid is a three-dimensional structure. This shape, which can change when a food is heated or cooked, and its pattern within a protein molecule determines if an adverse reaction will be triggered.

When an amino acid (protein component) in a food is identified as an allergen in an IgE-mediated reaction, IgE attaches itself to the amino acid and alerts the appropriate B cell. The B cell then sprays the amino acid with chemicals, usually histamine, and symptoms (diarrhea, hives, skin rash, wheezing, or worse) are experienced. Some foods, like peanuts, can cause a severe reaction because large numbers of mast cells throughout the body may be alerted and activated all at once. The result is a massive release of histamine at the same time with potentially fatal results.

ADVERSE FOOD REACTIONS—"TRUE" ALLERGY OR SOMETHING ELSE?

A food allergy is defined as an exaggerated immune response triggered by a specific food, usually a protein. There are different classification systems in use when defining food allergies and hypersensitivities. In the 1960s researchers Robin Coombs and P. H. G. Gell established the most widely used allergy classification system. This classification system, called the Gell and Coombs Classification System, defines six different classes of hypersensitive reactions. Type I hypersensitivity and Type IV hypersensitivity classes define adverse food reactions (Gell and Coombs, 1968). Type I hypersensitivity reactions occur when IgE antibodies are produced and mast cells or basophils release inflammatory mediators. Type IV hypersensitivity reactions are non-IgE adverse food reactions and are known as food intolerances.

In 2001 The European Academy of Allergology and Clinical Immunology (EAACI) proposed redefining an allergy as "a hypersensitivity reaction initiated by immunologic mechanisms" (Johansson, 2001). The EAACI distinguishes an adverse food reaction as a food hypersensitivity. Hypersensitivity is defined as "... objectively reproducible symptoms or signs, initiated by exposure to a defined stimulus at a dose tolerated by normal subjects" (Johansson, 2001) and is distinguished by whether IgE antibodies are produced or not. If IgE antibodies are produced, the reaction is classified as a food allergy or IgE-mediated food allergy. All other adverse food reactions, including food intolerances and food-related medical disorders or hypersensitivities, are classified as nonallergic food hypersensitivity. Because both classification systems are in use today, for clarity, the nomenclature used in the United States will be used here with the EAACI definitions in parentheses.

Type I hypersensitivity (food allergy) defines a "true" food allergy as a reaction that stimulates the immune system to produce IgE when an allergenic food is eaten. Termed IgE-mediated food allergy, food allergies are divided into two categories: immediate hypersensitivity reactions and delayed hypersensitivity reactions. Symptoms that develop anywhere from within minutes to one to two hours after eating the offending food are called immediate hypersensitivity reactions. In delayed hypersensitivity reactions, symptoms usually do not appear until twenty-four to seventy-two hours later and occur at the cellular level of the immune system (a Th2 response). True food allergies are relatively rare and account for only a small percentage of adverse food reactions, involving a limited number of foods.

Type IV hypersensitivity (nonallergic food hypersensitivity) defines all other adverse food reactions and is usually caused by food intolerances, food chemical reactions, or food-related medical disorders. There are different types

Lactose Intolerance Reaction

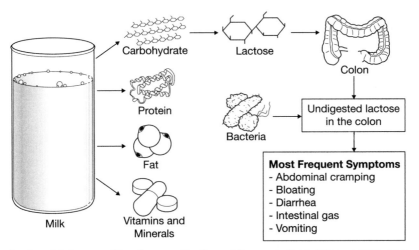

Lactose intolerance differs from a milk allergy. When an individual has an intolerance to the milk sugar lactose, the enzyme that is usually present to break it down for digestion is missing. Thus, lactose passes through the intestinal track undigested. Bacteria in the colon begin to work on the undigested lactose, producing some symptoms that mimic those caused by a milk allergy.

Figure 1.2. Lactose Intolerance Reaction [Jeff Dixon].

of nonallergic food hypersensitivity classifications: food intolerances (metabolic disorders), anaphylactoid reactions, and idiosyncratic reactions.

Food intolerances or metabolic food disorders are inborn defects in food metabolism. A very common worldwide example is lactose intolerance. Milk and dairy products contain lactose, a milk sugar. Many people lack the intestinal enzyme, β-galactosidase (also called lactase), which breaks down the lactose molecule. When this enzyme is missing, lactose remains intact as it travels through the intestine. Bacteria then begin to work on the undigested lactose when it reaches the colon. This bacterial action produces symptoms of abdominal pain, bloating, cramping, diarrhea, or intestinal gas. While some of these symptoms mimic milk allergy symptoms, milk intolerance is actually a defect in lactose digestion and *not* a "true" milk allergy.

An anaphylactoid reaction is a severe adverse reaction to an unidentified food substance. While this type of reaction is typically an adverse reaction to a pharmaceutical drug, some foods—primarily some fruits and vegetables—have been reported to trigger these types of reactions. Strawberries are one example of a food that can cause an anaphylactoid reaction. No specific allergen in strawberries has yet been discovered (although natural histamine levels in strawberries are suspected) nor do they contain protein. Yet some people experience anaphylaxis after eating strawberries for reasons still unknown.

Idiosyncratic reactions occur for unidentified reasons and are not "true" food allergies because they do not activate the immune system. The following, all of which will be explored in depth in a later chapter, can trigger adverse food reactions:

- Food additives
  - Aspartame
  - Benzoates
  - BHA (butylated hydroxyanisole)
  - BHT (butylated hydroxtoluene)
  - MSG (monosodium glutamate)
  - Nitrates and nitrites
  - Parabens
  - Sulfites
  - Tartrazine (FD&C yellow dye #5)
- Food poisoning
- Allergic intoxication:
  - Histamine poisoning
  - Tyramine sensitivity

- Medical disorders
  - Food intolerances
  - Eosinophil-associated gastrointestinal disorders (EGID)
  - Food-dependent exercise-induced anaphylaxis
  - Food protein-induced entercolitis or proctocolitis (allergic procto-colitis) syndrome
  - Gluten-sensitive enteropathy (gluten intolerance, celiac disease, celiac sprue)
  - Gustatory flushing syndrome
  - Heiner syndrome
  - Digestive and inflammatory bowel diseases
  - Oral allergy syndrome
  - Pseudofood allergy syndrome

As can be seen, adverse food reactions can be caused by a number of different triggers and can mimic food allergy symptoms. Take the case of four-year-old Wayne. His parents suspected he suffered from a food allergy. Whenever he ate strawberries, lemon-drop candy, corn chips with salsa, or chewed cinnamon gum, he would develop a bright red "rash" within minutes. This rash was not itchy and would quickly disappear, usually within a few minutes. No other symptoms occurred and the foods were not related in any way. Testing showed that his immune system was not involved and that his reaction was not an allergic response. Still believing he had a food allergy, his parents continued to severely restrict his diet. A visit to a trained food allergist, who reviewed all blood tests and took a careful medical history, uncovered the fact that Wayne actually had a medical disorder called gustatory flushing syndrome (Sicherer, 2006). This medical disorder triggers symptoms of red spots on the cheeks or blushing when tart or spicy foods are eaten. The tartness of the food activates a nerve in the cheek, which in turn causes blood vessels to dilate and stimulates excess salivation, causing symptoms. This adverse food reaction, classified as a Type IV hypersensitivity (nonallergic food hypersensitivity), does not necessitate unnecessary food restrictions. But this one example highlights that treatment varies for each of these triggers, and diets can be unnecessarily restricted without an accurate diagnosis. It is extremely important that a qualified physician make an accurate diagnosis of any adverse food-related symptoms for proper treatment and diet modifications.

2

Are Foods the Problem?

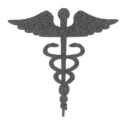

Most people assume they have a food allergy when they experience an adverse food reaction. In reality, only a small percentage of these (1–2 percent of adults and 5–7 percent of children) are "true" food allergies as confirmed by diagnosis. Incorrect assumptions about an adverse food reaction can lead to unnecessary food restrictions or incorrect treatment options. Diagnosing the problem isn't as easy as it might seem. While some symptoms strongly implicate a food and leave no doubt, some are much more subtle and similar to other food-related medical disorders or hypersensitivities. Seeking the help of a qualified health care professional is an important step toward identifying the problem and learning how to correctly treat it. Symptom overviews and methods used to diagnose food allergies and hypersensitivities are the focus of this chapter.

SYMPTOMS OF "TRUE" FOOD ALLERGIES

Symptoms of food allergies and hypersensitivities range from mild to severe and vary from person to person. Accurate diagnosis is especially difficult because there is no "typical" pattern of symptoms or way to predict the severity of a reaction. Consider the case of seven-year-old Erin (Sicherer, 2006), who is allergic to eggs and peanuts. Erin received medical care for four allergic reactions. During her first reaction, she vomited and developed hives. Her second reaction was severe with coughing, stomach pain, swelling in the throat, and wheezing. During her third reaction, she experienced hives only, and her fourth reaction was an itchy mouth accompanied by hives around the lips. Symptoms and their severity were different during each reaction she experienced.

Even though symptoms are difficult to predict, there are some universal symptoms that implicate food as a possible trigger, which are listed in Table 2.1. In general, adverse food reactions typically affect the digestive, respiratory, and/or skin systems. Severe, life-threatening reactions, such as anaphylaxis, always involve the circulatory and respiratory systems. Seeking an accurate diagnosis requires the skills of a trained allergist specializing in food allergies (not all are) and, sometimes, a gastroenterologist.

Table 2.1
Universal Symptoms of Food Allergy

Respiratory System
- Asthma
- Difficulty breathing
- Dry, raspy cough
- Earache
- Fainting
- Hoarseness, frequent throat clearing
- Itching or tightness in the throat or chest
- Paleness
- Runny nose

Circulatory System
- Chills
- Dizziness
- Fainting
- Heart attack
- Irregular heartbeat
- Paleness
- Sense of doom, panic
- Sudden weakness
- Weak pulse

Nervous System
- Dizziness
- Fatigue
- Hyperactivity
- Listlessness
- Migraines, frequent headaches

Digestive System
- Abdominal pain
- Belching
- Bloating
- Constipation
- Diarrhea
- Difficulty swallowing
- Indigestion
- Itchy mouth
- Metallic taste in mouth
- Nausea
- Vomiting

Circulatory and Respiratory Systems
Anaphylaxis:
- Dizziness
- Fainting
- Gastrointestinal symptoms
- Heart arrhythmias
- Heart attack
- Hives and angioedema
- Low blood pressure
- Respiratory symptoms
- Tunnel vision

So what symptoms should alert an individual to the fact that food may be the culprit? "True" food allergies usually affect the skin first. Symptoms of hives, eczema, or angioedema indicate a food may be the cause of an adverse reaction. Hives, also called urticaria, are extremely itchy, raised white areas surrounded by a reddened area on the skin. When an allergen triggers histamine release, which then permits fluid to leak out of blood vessels underneath the skin, hives occur. Appearing suddenly, and for no apparent reason, they are often assumed to be food related. But hives can also be caused by anxiety, chemical reactions (e.g., as a reaction to penicillin), extreme temperatures, irritations (e.g., clothes rubbing directly on the skin), or viruses. A food becomes a suspect when hives erupt within a few minutes to four hours after a food is eaten and there is no other obvious cause. If hives occur after four hours, it is more likely that food is not responsible for them.

Eczema, also known as atopic dermatitis, is a chronic skin condition identified by extremely dry and itchy skin. Although eczema may be caused by a large number of environmental triggers, approximately 40 percent of children with eczema also have a food allergy. Allergies to egg, milk, peanut, soy, and wheat have a strong link with eczema symptoms.

Angioedema, or swelling, can occur alone but usually accompanies hives. It often causes welts (especially around the eyes and on the face), swollen lips, intestinal swelling (causing a painful stomachache), and difficulty breathing. Anyone who has seen the movie "Hutch" will remember that Will Smith's character experienced facial swelling along with swollen ears, eyes, and lips after eating sushi—one classic example of angioedema.

The respiratory tract is also commonly affected by food allergies with symptoms of a stuffy or runny nose and swelling of the airway and/or bronchial tubes in the lungs, leading to asthma-like symptoms. All symptoms that affect the respiratory system can be life-threatening. Any external swelling, which is easily noted since it can be seen, can also be accompanied by unseen internal swelling. Internal swelling of the respiratory system is especially dangerous because symptoms may occur again a few hours after the initial reaction appears to be over. Therefore, *it is critical to seek immediate medical attention and be monitored for delayed reactions whenever the respiratory system is affected.*

Symptoms that affect the digestive tract are frequently assumed to be caused by a food allergy because all foods must pass through the digestive system, providing direct contact with a possible food allergen. But many food-related medical disorders or sensitivities can cause similar symptoms, making digestive tract symptoms caused by a "true" food allergy especially difficult to diagnosis. As a rule, gastrointestinal symptoms that are indicative of a "true" food allergy include:

Acute Symptoms	Abdominal pain
	Diarrhea
	Itchy mouth
	Nausea
	Tongue swelling
	Vomiting
Delayed Symptoms	Constipation (rare)
	Gastroesophageal reflux
	Persistent abdominal pain
	Weight loss or poor growth in children

Life-threatening reactions affect more than one body system and always involve the respiratory and circulatory systems (except in children, in which the circulatory system is not usually involved). Symptoms of anaphylaxis include dizziness, fainting, gastrointestinal symptoms, heart arrhythmias, heart attacks, hives and angioedema, low blood pressure, respiratory symptoms, and tunnel vision.

Ten to fifteen percent of food allergies occur in young children with a family history of allergies. If both parents have an allergy, which does not have to be a food allergy, their chance of having children who develop food allergies is two to three times greater than it is for children born into families with no history of allergies. Babies, infants, and young children are at the most risk for developing food allergies during the first two years of their life. Symptoms in susceptible children occur from within minutes up to two hours after eating a new food and include abdominal pain, dry or raspy cough, diarrhea, hives, itching or tightness in the throat, itchy eyes, nausea, rash or eczema, runny nose, shortness of breath, swelling of the lips, tongue, and face, vomiting, or wheezing or asthma.

Many food allergy sufferers and their families worry that they will underestimate the severity of symptoms and react too late. When judging symptoms and deciding if anaphylaxis is a potential threat, the following signs should always be evaluated:

1. Are skin symptoms present (hives, itch, flushing, swollen lips, tongue)?
2. Is the respiratory system compromised (difficulty breathing or a wheeze)?
3. Is the gastrointestinal system involved (abdominal pain or vomiting)?

An anaphylactic reaction is most likely imminent if two or more of these body systems are involved. Providing treatment and telephoning 911 emergency services should be immediately carried out. Determining what food was eaten, history of past reactions, and current symptoms also indicate how serious the reaction could become. Take the case of Jenny, a four-year-old allergic to milk (Sicherer, 2006). Jenny ate some of her brother's ice cream. Should she be given emergency treatment even though she may not have any or only mild symptoms? If she developed only hives and no other symptoms, then no treatment may be necessary. If she turned pale, cleared her throat, coughed, and vomited, immediate treatment should be given. But what if current symptoms are still mild but four previous reactions were severe, resulting in hospitalizations? In this case, treating her for anaphylaxis while symptoms are mild would be the prudent decision because the side effects of unnecessary medicine is minimal compared to the high risk of not treating her if symptoms quickly progress to a life-threatening level.

SYMPTOMS—OTHER CULPRITS

As noted before, symptoms of food allergies are frequently confused with those of food-related medical conditions or hypersensitivities because they are often similar. Because of this, Type IV hypersensitivities (nonallergic food hypersensitivity) can be very difficult and tricky to diagnose. As outlined in chapter 1, adverse food reactions can also be caused by:

- Food additives
- Food poisoning
- Allergic intoxications
- Medical disorders:
  - Food intolerances
  - Eosinophil-associated gastrointestinal disorders (EGID)
  - Food-dependent exercise-induced anaphylaxis
  - Food protein-induced entercolitis or proctocolitis (allergic proctocolitis) syndrome
  - Gluten-sensitive enteropathy (gluten intolerance, celiac disease, celiac sprue)
  - Gustatory flushing syndrome
  - Heiner syndrome
  - Digestive and inflammatory bowel diseases
  - Oral allergy syndrome
  - Pseudofood allergy syndrome

Diagnosis of these conditions is based on symptoms, negative food allergy test results, and other appropriate testing procedures. Each of these will be explored in-depth in the remainder of this chapter.

Food additives are defined by federal regulations as ". . . all substances . . ., the intended use of which results or may reasonably be expected to result, directly or indirectly, either in their becoming a component or otherwise affecting the characteristics of food" (FDA, 2003, online www.foodsafety.gov). Unless foods are grown, harvested, and cooked or canned by individual consumers, many packaged and convenience foods (and many cosmetics, medications, and toiletries) contain additives that decrease the risk of food spoilage, preserve and enhance flavor, or improve the physical appearance of a food. Salting, smoking, pickling or canning vegetables with vinegar, and adding herbs, spices, sugar, minerals, vitamins, or other nutrients to foods has been a common practice for many centuries. Archeological evidence discovered Ancient Egyptians preserved food by drying, salting, and fermenting foods for later use. Foods were colored by using saffron and the crushed insect Coccus cacti (a parasite living on cacti, which were crushed to make a carmine or reddish purple dye capable of triggering an anaphylactic reaction). Gum arabic (a natural gum from the sap of the acacia tree) was used to thicken and emulsify liquids.

More than 3,000 ingredients have been approved for use as food additives in the United States, and each approved additive undergoes safety reviews prior to approval for use. Some of these additives occur naturally, but many are synthetically made. In 1903 the Bureau of Chemistry (known as the Food and Drug Administration [FDA] today) established safety standards for chemical preservatives used in medications and foods through the volunteer efforts of the "Poison Squad." The Poison Squad, a group of young men who volunteered to eat only foods that had been treated with measured amounts of chemical preservatives, served as human guinea pigs to study the safety and side effects of food preservatives used at the time. Known poisons were prohibited. But the safety of many chemical additives still remained unknown, even today long after their volunteer efforts were over. Passage of the Pesticide Amendment (1954), the Food Additives Amendment (1958), and the Color Additive Amendments (1960) drastically changed the way food manufacturers operated and for the first time required them to evaluate all new food ingredients before adding them into foods. Today, food additives allowed for use in the United States are classified as "Generally Recognized As Safe" (GRAS) substances.

The European Food Safety Authority (EFSA) evaluates and regulates food additives in the European Union. The Joint Expert Committee on Food Additives (JECFA), administered by both the Food and Agriculture Organization (FAO) and the World Health Organization (WHO), evaluates food additives on the international level. This joint effort develops General Standards for Food Additives (GSFA) on a global basis. Their efforts have also produced a database of approved substances called the Codex alimentarius, which is

Table 2.2
Common Food Additives

The following summary lists the types of common food ingredients, why they are used, and some examples of the names that can be found on product labels. Some additives are used for more than one purpose.

Ingredients	What They Do	Examples of Uses	Names Found on Product Labels
Preservatives	Prevent food spoilage from bacteria, molds, fungi, or yeast (antimicrobials); slow or prevent changes in color, flavor, or texture and delay rancidity (antioxidants); maintain freshness	Fruit sauces and jellies, beverages, baked goods, cured meats, oils and margarines, cereals, dressings, snack foods, fruits and vegetables	Ascorbic acid, citric acid, sodium benzoate, calcium propionate, sodium erythorbate, sodium nitrite, calcium sorbate, potassium sorbate, BHA, BHT, EDTA, tocopherols (Vitamin E)
Sweeteners	Add sweetness with or without the extra calories	Beverages, baked goods, confections, table-top sugar, substitutes, many processed foods	Sucrose (sugar), glucose, fructose, sorbitol, mannitol, corn syrup, high fructose corn syrup, saccharin, aspartame, sucralose, acesulfame potassium (acesulfame-K), neotame
Color Additives	Offset color loss due to exposure to light, air, temperature extremes, moisture and storage conditions; correct natural variations in color; enhance colors that occur naturally; provide color to colorless and "fun" foods	Many processed foods (candies, snack foods, margarine, cheese, soft drinks, jams/jellies, gelatins, pudding and pie fillings)	FD&C Blue Nos. 1 and 2, FD&C Green No. 3, FD&C Red Nos. 3 and 40, FD&C Yellow No. 5 (tartrazine) and No. 6, Orange B, Citrus Red No. 2, annatto extract, beta-carotene, grape skin extract, cochineal extract or carmine, paprika oleoresin, caramel color, fruit and vegetable juices, saffron (Note: Exempt color additives are not required to be declared by name on labels but may be declared simply as colorings or color added)

(continued)

Table 2.2 (continued)

Ingredients	What They Do	Examples of Uses	Names Found on Product Labels
Flavors and Spices	Add specific flavors (natural and synthetic)	Pudding and pie fillings, gelatin dessert mixes, cake mixes, salad dressings, candies, soft drinks, ice cream, BBQ sauce	Natural flavoring, artificial flavor, spices
Flavor Enhancers	Enhance flavors already present in foods (without providing their own separate flavor)	Many processed foods	Monosodium glutamate (MSG), hydrolyzed soy protein, autolyzed yeast extract, disodium guanylate or inosinate
Fat Replacers (and components of formulations used to replace fats)	Provide expected texture and a creamy "mouth-feel" in reduced-fat foods	Provide expected texture and a creamy "mouth-feel" in reduced-fat foods	Olestra, cellulose gel, carrageenan, polydextrose, modified food starch, micro-particulated egg white protein, guar gum, xanthan gum, whey protein concentrate
Nutrients	Replace vitamins and minerals lost in processing (enrichment), add nutrients that may be lacking in the diet (fortification)	Flour, breads, cereals, rice, macaroni, margarine, salt, milk fruit beverages, energy bars, instant breakfast drinks	Thiamine hydrochloride, riboflavin (Vitamin B2), niacin, niacinamide, folate or folic acid, beta carotene, potassium iodide, iron or ferrous sulfate, alpha tocopherols, ascorbic acid, vitamin D, amino acids (L-tryptophan, L-lysine, L-leucine, L-methionine)

Type of Additive	Function	Found in	Examples
Emulsifiers	Allow smooth mixing of ingredients, prevent separation, keep emulsified products stable, reduce stickiness, control crystallization, keep ingredients dispersed, and help products dissolve more easily	Salad dressings, peanut butter, chocolate, margarine, frozen desserts	Soy lecithin, mono- and diglycerides, egg yolks, polysorbates, sorbitan monostearate
Stabilizers and Thickeners, Binders, Texturizers	Produce uniform texture, improve "mouth-feel"	Frozen desserts, dairy products, cakes, pudding and gelatin mixes, dressings, jams and jellies, sauces	Gelatin, pectin, guar gum, carrageenan, xanthan gum, whey
Leavening Agents	Promote rising of baked goods	Breads and other baked goods	Baking soda, monocalcium phosphate, calcium carbonate
Anti-caking agents	Keep powdered foods free-flowing, prevent moisture absorption	Salt, baking powder, confectioner's sugar	Calcium silicate, iron ammonium citrate, silicon dioxide
Humectants	Retain moisture	Shredded coconut, marshmallows, soft candies, confections	Glycerin, sorbitol
Yeast Nutrients	Promote growth of yeast	Breads and other baked goods	Calcium sulfate, ammonium phosphate
Dough Strengtheners and Conditioners	Produce more stable dough	Breads and other baked goods	Ammonium sulfate, azodicarbonamide, L-cysteine
Firming Agents	Maintain crispness and firmness	Processed fruits and vegetables	Calcium chloride, calcium lactate
Enzyme Preparations	Modify proteins, polysaccharides and fats	Cheese, dairy products, meat	Enzymes, lactase, papain, rennet, chymosin
Gases	Serve as propellant, aerate, or create carbonation	Oil cooking spray, whipped cream, carbonated beverages	Carbon dioxide, nitrous oxide

Source: Reprinted with permission from the International Food Information Council Foundation (IFIC) and the Food and Drug Administration (FDA), March 2005 (September 2008), http://www.ific.org.

available at their Web site, http://www.codexalimentarius.net/gsfaonline/index.html.

Despite testing and general consensus that these substances are safe for use in foods, some food additives are known to cause hypersensitivity or allergic reactions in sensitive individuals. These reactions have been classified as food intolerances (nonallergic food hypersensitivities) rather than allergies because the immune system is not activated. Although rare, food additives that are most frequently reported to trigger adverse reactions in sensitive individuals are listed below.

- Aspartame
- Benzoates
- BHA (butylated hydroxyanisole)
- BHT (butylated hydroxtoluene)
- Gelatin
- MSG (monosodium glutamate)
- Nitrates and nitrites
- Parabens
- Sorbate and sorbic acid
- Sulfites
- Tartrazine (FD&C yellow dye #5)

All have been reported to cause adverse reactions in sensitive individuals, but aspartame, benzoates, MSG, sulfites, and the natural preservative gelatin are some of the more notable.

Aspartame, a low-calorie sweetener widely used in foods or beverages, is sold under the brand names NutraSweet® and Equal®. Phenylalanine and aspartic acid, two amino acids the body uses to make protein, are combined together to make aspartame. Phenylalanine is found naturally in protein-rich foods such as beans, eggs, fish, ice cream, milk, poultry, nuts, and red meats. Trace amounts are found in bread, cereals, cookies, some fruits and vegetables, pasta, and rice. Babies born with a genetic disorder, diagnosed as phenylketonuria (PKU), cannot metabolize phenylalanine. Therefore, it is imperative that all dietary sources of PKU be eliminated from their diet or brain damage will occur. Aspartic acid occurs naturally in grapefruit, nectarines, oranges, plums, prunes, and strawberries. Many juice concentrates also tend to be high in it.

When phenylalanine and aspartic acid are eaten via natural food sources, their digestion and absorption are at a pace the body safely manages, but when they are ingested via aspartame, digestion and absorption occur rapidly. Although a rare occurrence, some individuals do experience symptoms after eating aspartame that include abdominal cramps, bloating, diarrhea, difficulty in concentrating, eczema, headache, hives, irritability, joint and muscle aches, nasal stuffiness, and wheezing, among others.

Benzoates are chemicals used as preservatives to prevent the growth of bacteria, fungus, and yeast. Sodium and potassium benzoate use is widespread in beverages, cosmetics, foods, medicines, mouthwashes, nutritional supplements, and toothpastes. Benzoates have been found to change into the carcinogen benzene when they interact with vitamin C (ascorbic acid) or are exposed to high temperatures. The World Health Organization (WHO) noted in a 2000 report that, "In humans, the acute toxicity of benzoic acid and sodium benzoate is low. However, both substances are known to cause non-immunological contact reactions (pseudoallergy)" (WHO, 2000). Symptoms of benzoate sensitivity include angioedema, asthma, headache, hives, and vomiting.

Monosodium glutamate (MSG) is a flavoring agent used in many processed and cooked foods and is also called hydrolyzed protein or protein hydrolysate. When one molecule of glutamic acid (an amino acid) is added to one molecule of sodium, it creates the molecule MSG. Most people are familiar with MSG because it is a regularly added ingredient in many Chinese dishes and can have a negative interaction with some cardiovascular medications. Every plant and animal cell makes MSG naturally, and it is a common substance in foods, such as cheese, milk, meat, mushrooms, and peas. Like aspartame, the MSG molecule is rapidly broken down and absorbed by the body. However, large quantities may overwhelm the body because it cannot be absorbed quickly, causing symptoms of abdominal cramps, bloating, diarrhea, difficulty concentrating, eczema, headache, hives, irritability, joint and muscle aches, stuffy nose, and wheezing. MSG has been linked to hives, neurological diseases such as Alzheimer's, neurotoxicity (damage to nerves), and weight gain, although more research is needed in these areas.

Sulfite-induced asthma is caused by sulfites, a preservative used to prevent browning, to provide a bleaching effect in foods, or as a preservative in some pharmaceutical medications. It has been reported by sensitive individuals to cause abdominal pain, chest pain, cramping, diarrhea, difficulty swallowing, fainting, headache, hives, itching, loss of consciousness, nausea, rashes, swelling, vomiting, and changes in body temperature and heart rate. For some, sulfites can induce life-threatening asthma. Sulfites are added to numerous foods, as well as occurring naturally in foods. They are considered a chemical sensitivity because testing methods do not confirm an allergic immune response. Avoiding sulfites usually prevents symptoms.

Gelatin is a natural food additive derived from egg protein (used in many vaccines), beef, pork, and sometimes fish. In some allergic individuals it has been reported to cause food allergy symptoms, although this is a rare occur-rence. Gelatin is also included in some candies, desserts, and yogurts. If a sen-sitive individual has an allergy to any of these foods, they should avoid gelatin and discuss vaccine alternatives with their doctors.

Food poisoning is an illness caused by eating foods or drinks that are conta-minated with bacteria, parasites, viruses, metals, prions, or toxins. Although it is *not* a food hypersensitivity or allergy, mild symptoms can be confused with them. Symptoms almost always affect the gastrointestinal system and usually occur from two to six hours after eating or drinking the infected food or liquid. Abdominal cramps, bloating, diarrhea, nausea, or vomiting are usually the first signs of food poisoning. Symptoms and their severity depend on the microor-ganism contaminating the food or drink source. Some microorganisms or tox-ins can produce severe symptoms that include confusion, numbness, tingling of face, hands, and feet, and weakness. The Medline Plus Medical Encyclope-dia of the National Library of Medicine and the National Institutes of Health provides specific information about the types of different microorganisms that may cause food poisoning, which may be accessed on their Web site at http://www.nlm.nih.gov/medlineplus/ency/article/001652.htm.

Emergency room doctors usually distinguish food poisoning from a food allergy by the length of time it takes for symptoms to appear. Although onset can range anywhere from half an hour to six months, depending on the micro-organism and body system affected, symptoms of most cases of food poisoning usually appear within twelve hours after ingestion. Symptoms of a food allergy appear within five minutes to two hours after eating, and symptoms of food hypersensitivity become distinguishable when they appear every time a specific food is eaten and not as an infrequent occurrence, as is usually the case with food poisoning.

Allergic intoxications include histamine poisoning and tyramine sensitivity. Histamine poisoning, also known as scombroid poisoning, is caused by foods containing histamine. Histamine, naturally present in fermented foods such as bologna, bratwurst, cheese, kefir, pepperoni, salami, sausages, smoked and pick-led meats, tofu, and yogurt, can also be found in eggplant, spinach, strawber-ries, and tomatoes. The effect of histamine in foods may be intensified when eaten with, or combined with, alcohol, egg whites, shellfish, and strawberries. Food and medication dyes, like tartrazine, and preservatives, like benzoates, can also trigger mast cells to release histamine as well.

Scombroid fish, which includes anchovies, bonito, butterfly kingfish, herring, kahawai, mackeral, marlin, pilchards, salmon, sardines, swordfish, and tuna, is the most frequent reason for scrombroid poisoning when it is improperly handled and stored. The amino acid histidine is present in the gastrointestinal tract of scombroid fish. After these fish are caught, bacteria in the intestine begin to convert histidine into histamine. This conversion happens quickly if the fish is not properly gutted or chilled. Freezing or cooking does not kill this toxin. Symptoms of histamine poisoning usually occur within thirty minutes to a few hours after eating contaminated fish and include a tingling or peppery sensation in the mouth, burning or itching of the skin, diarrhea, faintness, headache, nausea, a rash on the upper body, and vomiting.

A hypersensitivity reaction to tyramine, an amino acid used to regulate blood pressure and derived from tyrosine that is found naturally in the body, can also cause adverse food reactions in some individuals. Tyramine is found in avocados, bananas, beer, aged cheeses, chicken livers, chocolate, some drugs, eggplant, fava beans, figs, gravies, plums, raspberries, red plums, sour cream, soy sauce, tomatoes, vinegars, wine (especially red), and yeast extracts. Symptoms of tyramine hypersensitivity include hives and/or migraine headaches.

Although there are some medical disorders that are speculated to be triggered by foods (Table 2.3), research has no conclusive evidence to date that firmly links them. However, other medical disorders known as food intolerances (nonallergic food hypersensitivity) have evidence showing a connection to food triggers. Most food intolerances are actually caused by an inborn defect in food digestion and metabolism and include lactose, fructose, and gluten intolerances. Lactose intolerance, a common digestive defect worldwide, affects about 70 percent of the world population and is often confused with milk allergy. Symptoms of a milk allergy will usually occur immediately after consuming milk or milk products. Typical symptoms involve the immune system and include bloating, diarrhea, gas, hives, vomiting, wheezing, and the possibility of anaphylactic shock. But some of these symptoms are very similar to those of lactose intolerance. Symptoms of lactose intolerance include abdominal cramping, bloating, diarrhea, and gas. Distinguishing between the two is based on results of allergy testing, symptoms, and results of a lactose tolerance test, hydrogen breath test, and, in young children or infants, a stool acidity test.

Infants are usually born with adequate amounts of the enzyme lactase, which breaks down the milk sugar lactose that is naturally present in milk and milk products. After maturity, lactose begins to decline in the adult gastrointestinal tract. For some people, this decline is significant enough to allow lactose to pass undigested through the colon, where bacteria begins to work on it. This bacterial action produces symptoms listed above, but lactose intolerance does not activate the immune system and can be a temporary condition. Normal gastrointestinal flora can be destroyed with antibiotic use and by some cancer treatments. When these medications or treatments are over, the normal gastrointestinal flora returns and with it, sometimes, the ability to digest lactose again.

Table 2.3
Suspected Food Associations with Some Medical Disorders

Medical Condition	Common Suspected Food Triggers
Arthritis	Alcohol
	Caffeine
	Chocolate
	Citrus fruit
	Dairy products
	Eggs
	Fish
	Gluten
	Meat
	Nightshade vegetables (cayenne pepper, eggplant, ground cherries, huckleberry, paprika, sweet and hot peppers, pimentos, potatoes, tabasco sauce, tomatoes)
	Poultry
	Sugar
Asthma	Aspartame
	Aspirin (salicylates)
	Avocado
	Banana
	Benzoate/benzoic acid
	BHA/BHT
	Citrus fruits
	Cow's milk
	Eggs
	Fish
	MSG
	Nitrites
	Peanuts
	Potatoes
	Shellfish
	Soy
	Sulfites
	Tartrazine and other food dyes
	Tomatoes
	Tree nuts
	Wheat

Table 2.3 (continued)

Medical Condition	Common Suspected Food Triggers
Attention-Deficit Hyperactivity Disorder (ADHD)	Individual allergies to specific foods and sensitivities to specific food additives
Dermatitis	Azo dyes (used in clothes, food, drugs)
	Benzoates
	Berries
	Citrus
	Cow's milk
	Eggs
	Fish
	Gluten
	Peanuts
	Shellfish
	Soy
	Sulfites
	Tree nuts
	Wheat
Migraines	Alcoholic beverages
	Apples
	Aspartame
	Beer
	Chocolate
	Citrus fruits
	Corn
	Eggs, nuts, tomatoes
	Gluten
	Meat, fish, poultry
	Milk and dairy products
	MSG
	Nitrites
	Onions
	Peanuts
	Tyramine
	Wheat
	Wine

Fructose intolerance is similar to lactose intolerance, but there are two distinct forms of defective fructose metabolism. The first, hereditary fructose intolerance (HFI), is a rare medical disorder of fructose metabolism caused by a deficiency of the enzyme aldolase B. Aldolase B facilitates the breakdown of fructose. When fructose cannot be broken down, it accumulates in the liver, kidney, and small intestine. Symptoms include severe abdominal pain, severe hypoglycemia, vomiting, and eventually liver or kidney failure causing death. The second medical disorder, fructose malabsorption (FM), is the incomplete absorption of fructose in the small intestine and often confused with HFI. When fructose is malabsorbed, intestinal bacteria work on it, producing symptoms that include abdominal pain, bloating, altered bowel patterns, gas, and lack of energy. Fructose is a simple sugar found naturally in fruits, honey, and some baked products and vegetables. High fructose corn syrup (HFCS), a very controversial food additive, is an extremely common additive in many processed foods. Enzymatic assays of aldolase activity from a liver biopsy and a fructose tolerance test are used to diagnosis HFI. A breath hydrogen test taken after ingesting fructose is used to diagnosis FM.

Gluten intolerance, also called gluten-sensitive enteropathy, celiac disease, celiac sprue, nontropical sprue, and idiopathic steatorrhea, is an inability to break down the wheat protein gliadin found in gluten. This intolerance will be discussed in more detail later in this chapter.

Eosinophil-associated gastrointestinal disorders (EGID) include eosinophilic colitis, esophagitis (also called allergic eosinophilic esophagitis [AEE]), gastritis, gastroenteritis (also called allergic eosinophilic gastroenteritis [AEG]), and enteritis. Eosinophils, white blood cells that become activated in response to infections and allergies, normally line the digestive tract. However, in these disorders they increase and accumulate abnormally along the digestive tract for unknown reasons, although elevated blood levels of IgE antibodies have been observed. In eosinophilic esophagitis (EE), eosinophils accumulate in the esophagus. In eosinophilic gastritis (EG), they accumulate in the stomach. In eosinophilic gastroenteritis and enteritis, they accumulate in the stomach and the small intestine. In eosinophilic colitis (EC), they accumulate in the colon or rectum. All EGIDs interfere with normal digestion and cause damage to the digestive tract. They can occur at any age, but EE is more common in adults and diagnosis is usually made during late childhood or the early teens. Symptoms include chronic abdominal or chest pain, bloating, blood in the stool and anemia, delayed growth in children, delayed stomach emptying after a meal, diarrhea, difficulty swallowing, food impactions (food that lodges in the throat), nausea and vomiting after eating, poor appetite, projectile vomiting in infants, reflux that does not respond to medications, difficulty sleeping, and weight loss. Diagnosis is made by using an endoscope to look at the lining of the gastrointestinal tract and taking tissue biopsies. If an EGID diagnosis is confirmed, food allergy testing is recommended because food allergies appear to play a role in EGID onset.

Food-dependent exercise-induced anaphylaxis (EIA) affects only a small percentage of people, who experience symptoms ranging from a rash to life-threatening anaphylaxis, when they exercise after eating a specific food. A very rare form of an allergic response, symptoms typically occur one to four hours after eating a trigger food *and* after any kind of physical exertion. However, if the person exercises without eating that particular food or eats that food and does not exercise, no adverse reaction will occur. Individuals with this disorder usually have a family history of asthma, hay fever, or chronic hives. Some pharmaceutical medications taken before physical activity can also trigger symptoms. Exercising within two to four hours after eating a specific food may cause hives and itching over the entire body, reddened skin, or swelling that progresses to life-threatening anaphylaxis without treatment.

There are three types of EIA: specific food EIA, nonspecific food EIA, and medication- or drug-dependent EIA. Specific food EIA is triggered by a combination of eating a specific food and physical activity. Nonspecific food EIA has yet to be linked to any one food and eating any food prior to exercise triggers it. Medication- or drug-dependent EIA develops after taking a specific medication followed by exercise. Drug-dependent EIA is associated with use of antibiotics, aspirin, cold remedies, and nonsteroidal anti-inflammatory drugs (NSAIDs). Foods that are reported to trigger EIA include celery, cheese, chickpeas, eggs, grapes, oysters, peaches, peas, pears, pizza, poppy seeds, shrimp, snails, and wheat. EIA typically affects athletes, especially in hot, humid, or cold weather, and allergy-sensitive individuals. However, no genetic pattern is apparent and it can affect anyone.

Food protein-induced entercolitis or proctocolitis (allergic proctocolitis) syndrome is seen in infants, usually before three months of age, and in children. Symptoms are bright red blood in the stool and prolonged projectile vomiting that begins one to three hours after drinking cow's milk or a soy protein-based formula. However, a connection has also been made with allergies to corn, eggs, fish, nuts, shellfish, and wheat. Breast-fed babies who are susceptible can develop this disorder when their mother eats any of these foods because the allergenic proteins pass through breast milk to the baby. When the allergenic protein is eliminated from the diet, symptoms usually resolve within forty-eight to seventy-two hours. Infants tend to outgrow this allergy by their first birthday. When it occurs in adults, which is rare, allergies to shellfish trigger it. Symptoms in adults include abdominal cramps, severe nausea, and prolonged vomiting, which develop within one to six hours after eating shellfish.

Gluten-sensitive enteropathy (celiac disease, celiac sprue, or gluten intolerance) is an inherited disease that affects the small intestine and is frequently confused with a wheat allergy. Although the immune system is involved, it is considered an autoimmune disease and *not* a food allergy because chemical mediators are not released in response to the presence of gluten found in wheat. Eating gluten, which contains the protein gliadin, triggers the immune system to attack this protein. Damage to the inner lining of the intestine results, leading to malabsorption of nutrients and subsequent medical disorders. Damage is reversible as long as gluten in the diet is strictly eliminated. Symptoms include abdominal pain, bloating, constipation or diarrhea, irritability, poor growth in children, and vomiting. Occasionally, symptoms of blistering skin rashes, poor bone development, and poorly developed tooth enamel are subtle signs of this disorder along with or instead of gastrointestinal symptoms. Diagnosis is made with blood tests and biopsies of the small intestine. Unlike some allergies, it cannot be outgrown, is associated with cancer, and has no other treatment than strict gluten avoidance. When diagnosed with this disease, it is important to eat a diet *containing* gluten *before* testing. Eliminating gluten from the diet prior to testing can cause a false-negative result.

Gustatory flushing syndrome (also called auriculotemporal syndrome and Frey's syndrome) is triggered by eating highly flavored foods, such as some lollipops or candies, spicy foods, tomatoes, and tangy or sour foods. These foods activate the auriculotemporal nerves, which control salivary and sweat glands and blood vessels in the face. These nerves cause facial blood vessels to dilate and excess salivation. Facial flushing or blushing or red spots on the cheeks are typical symptoms. This condition is harmless and disappears quickly. Various medications and surgeries have been tried, but with little success and undesirable side effects. Thus, it is best to avoid these foods and wait out any symptoms.

Heiner syndrome (HS) is a rare disorder with few documented cases and is a variation of the pulmonary disease hemosiderosis. HS, which occurs most often in children between the ages of six months and two years (although it can manifest itself at any age), is a hypersensitivity reaction to the proteins in cow's milk. Symptoms are usually anorexia, colic or diarrhea, chronic cough, fever, nasal congestion or runny nose, poor weight gain, recurrent ear infections, vomiting, or wheezing. Eliminating cow's milk and milk products from the diet usually resolves all symptoms. Diagnosis is made by using blood test results, symptoms, and lung X-rays.

Digestive and inflammatory bowel diseases include diverticulosis, diverticulitis, and irritable bowel syndrome (IBS). These digestive diseases sometimes involve a sensitivity or intolerance to a food. Ulcerative colitis and Crohn's disease are inflammatory bowel diseases (IBD) that are difficult to diagnose and often confused with food allergies or hypersensitivities. Diverticulosis and diverticulitis affect the large intestine (colon), and symptoms include abdominal cramping, bloating, constipation, diarrhea, and gas. Diverticulosis results when intestinal diverticula, small pouches that develop at weak spots along the colon, occur. Diverticulitis results when intestinal diverticula become infected. This condition is the most serious because the intestine can become perforated and peritonitis can develop, which is fatal if left untreated. Symptoms of diverticulitis also include fever, intestinal obstruction, nausea, severe abdominal pain, and vomiting. Both are diagnosed on the basis of symptoms, barium X-rays, and colonoscopy. Irritable bowel syndrome (IBS), also a digestive disease, is triggered by sensitivities to some foods, among other things. There are two types of IBS. IBS-C has the primary symptom of constipation, and IBS-D has the primary symptom of diarrhea. Other symptoms include abdominal pain, bloating, gas, and unpredictable bowel movements. It appears that food intolerance or disruption of normal intestinal bacterial flora may cause IBS. IBS has not been associated with more serious digestive diseases.

Ulcerative colitis affects the large intestine, and Crohn's disease affects both the small and large intestines. Diagnosis is made by blood tests and biopsies of the intestines. Symptoms for both IBDs include loss of appetite, frequent bowel movements, severe cramping, bloody diarrhea, fatigue, fever, and weight loss. Both Crohn's disease and ulcerative colitis show immune system abnormalities and some food sensitivities. But foods do not cause these disorders and treatment options do not involve food avoidance unless there is secondary food hypersensitivity or intolerance. The bacteria, *Mycobacterium paratuberculosis* (traced to milk from infected dairy cows), may play a role in these two medical disorders. One study found 65 percent of Crohn's disease patients tested positive for this bacteria, whereas only 4 percent of other IBDs tested positive for it (Melina, 2004).

Oral allergy syndrome (pollen-related allergy or cross-reactivity) occurs when the body confuses a specific food protein from one source with the same protein found in a different source. For instance, someone who is allergic to a protein in tree pollen may have an allergic reaction to the same protein also found in apples or cherries. An allergy to ragweed can cause a cross-reactivity reaction with bananas or cantaloupes. Allergies to latex rubber have been known to trigger severe anaphylactic reactions, but symptoms are usually mild and include mild lip swelling or itchy ears, lips, or mouth. These proteins are usually destroyed very easily by stomach acid, digestion, and cooking. For most of the food-related pollen allergens, an individual may experience an allergic reaction to the raw form of a food (raw apple) but not to the cooked form (apple juice, applesauce, etc.). Diagnosis of this disorder is made by using food allergy-testing methods (described later in this chapter). The following is a

Pollen	Food Cross-Reactivity
Birch	Apple, apricot, carrot, celery, cherry, hazelnut, kiwi, peach, plum, potato, pumpkin seed, strawberry, zucchini
Dust mites	Snails
Grass	Melon, peach, tomato
Latex	Avocado, banana, chestnuts, kiwi, mango, peach
Mugwort	Celery, chamomile, honey, tomato
Ragweed	Banana, melon, watermelon

partial listing of foods that cross-react with pollens. Other foods, mostly fruits and vegetables, may also cross-react and cause symptoms.

Pseudofood allergy syndrome is a disorder that usually affects adults who diagnose themselves, or have been misdiagnosed, and are convinced their symptoms are a food allergy. The only way to treat this syndrome is to correctly diagnose symptoms and treat any diagnosed medical disorders or hypersensitivities. While many of these individuals complain they are not taken seriously or have an underlying psychological component involved, it is important to realize that they may actually have a physical disorder that causes symptoms. One study of patients with chronic urticaria found an impaired permeability of the gastrointestinal tract, thus allowing potential allergens to pass into the bloodstream and triggering symptoms (Buhner, 2004). In the absence of any physical or medical reason for symptoms, education and counseling become important tools to use when discovering the root cause of symptoms.

MAKING THE CORRECT DIAGNOSIS

Diagnosing food allergies or hypersensitivities is tricky. There are many tests that claim to diagnose them, but to correctly diagnose an adverse food reaction, a qualified allergist who is specifically trained in food allergies and, occasionally, a gastroenterologist is needed. A general practitioner or internist is able to diagnose medical conditions but may miss the more subtle symptoms of a food-related problem that a food allergist frequently sees. Before visiting an allergist, it is extremely helpful to keep a careful record of symptoms. Recording symptoms in a notebook or using a form such as the one outlined in

Table 2.4 for three consecutive days (two weekdays and one weekend day should be included) should answer the following questions:

- What foods or drinks were consumed when symptoms occurred?
- Where was the food prepared (at home or eaten out)?
- How much was eaten?
- Where was the food eaten (at home, a restaurant, or outside)?
- How much time passed between when the food was eaten and the first symptom occurred?
- What were the symptoms?
- In what order did the symptoms appear?
- What symptoms usually occur and how did these differ from them?
- How were symptoms treated?
- How long did it take for the symptoms to go away?
- Were any prescription medicines or over-the-counter drugs taken before the reaction occurred?
- Was alcohol used before the reaction?
- What activity was performed before symptoms occurred (exercising, taking a shower, brushing teeth, etc.)?
- Have there been any recent changes at home (a new pet, new home furnishings, new home, etc.)?

All condiments (jams, mayonnaise, sugar, etc.), nutritional supplements, or medications should also be listed. It is especially important to be honest about the foods eaten and personal habits so an accurate diagnosis can be made as quickly as possible.

When seeing an allergist, a medical history, physical exam, and blood and skin tests will be completed first. The allergist will also ask if there is a family history of allergies and what they are. Serum IgE concentration, which checks the blood for the presence of IgE antibodies, will be evaluated. But high levels of IgE do not necessarily mean a food allergy. A second blood test, known as the RAST or radioallergosorbent test, will be taken and is regarded as one of the most accurate tests used to make a food-related diagnosis. This blood test drops blood onto a disk that contains specific food proteins. The disk is then measured for levels of antibodies that the blood produces. Different labs measure amounts of allergen-specific antibodies differently. However, testing methods are unpredictable. The higher the RAST score the more likely there is a possible allergy to that specific food protein. The RAST does not indicate a food allergy beyond a shadow of a doubt, though. Between 50 and 60 percent of positive RAST scores are actually false positives, and 10–30 percent of children have a food allergy even when their RAST score is negative. This means

Table 2.4
Food Reaction Self-Assessment Form
Keep a detailed record of symptoms, activities, and foods/liquids eaten:

Symptom/ Time Occurred	Food or Drink & Brand Name	Amount	Activity	Food Prep/Eaten	Treatment/Time Resolved
Example: Hives/ 10 minutes after lunch	**Example:** Peanut butter (Skippy®) Wheat bread (Pepperidge Farm®) 2% milk (Hood)	**Example:** 1 Tablespoon 2 slices 8 ounces	**Example:** Walked 30 min. before lunch	**Example:** Home/kitchen table	**Example:** Benadryl/1 hour

Medications:_____

Changes in environment:_____

that, while the test may indicate antibodies produced against a specific food allergen are present, it still does not indicate conclusive results.

Because foods have similar makeups within related food groups, the RAST may also react to the same allergen found in different foods within the group. For example, peanuts are in the legume food group. A positive RAST to peanuts can also be positive to other legumes, such as green beans. But an individual may have a reaction to peanuts and not green beans, even though the RAST tests positive for both. Or the individual may have a reaction to the raw food only and not react to the purified food extract used during the test. This could occur because the commercial food extract has been degraded because of a heating process and the individual is now able to tolerate it. CAP-RAST, ELISA (enzyme-linked immunosorbent assay), and ImmunoCAP blood tests are some test variations that may be used instead of the RAST. These also measure allergen antibody production and are reliable testing methods. Although blood tests are not conclusive, they are useful because they measure changes in IgE antibody production over time and can indicate if, in the case of children, a child is outgrowing a specific allergy or not. But blood tests are only one step in the process toward making a correct diagnosis.

Skin tests are the next step and are well liked as a diagnostic tool because they show immediate results, are inexpensive, and produce fewer false positives. It is important that oral antihistamine medications are stopped for about two weeks prior to testing, or test results may be inaccurate. Skin tests may also cause anaphylactic reactions, although this rarely happens. Some skin disorders, chronic conditions, and long-term use of corticosteroid medications can affect results. Skin tests are not recommended for those suffering from eczema, who experience delayed symptoms, or have cancer, diabetes, chronic renal failure, or spinal cord injuries.

There are three different types of skin tests used. In a skin prick test, a small, two-prong needle or plastic probe is used to "inject or plant" a small amount of a specific diluted and purified food extract solution directly under the top layer of skin on the back or forearm. In a scratch test, the skin is lightly scraped and the food extract dropped on the site. In an intradermal test, the food extract is injected just under the skin with a needle. A drop of salt water (saline) is also "planted" for use as a comparison site.

Occasionally, histamine will be used instead of saline. The number of sites planted vary according to age and allergens tested. Fewer skin prick tests are needed for infants and very young children because they are less likely to be sensitized to as many allergens as older children and adults. Suspected food allergies can vary from less than twenty to as many as eighty, depending on symptoms and whether they are inhaled or oral allergens. If oral allergy syndrome is suspected, a prick + prick test will be used. In this test, the needle will be dipped in the fresh fruit or vegetable, rather than an extract, because extracts are heated (and the protein subsequently broken down), which then may cause a false-negative reaction.

Positive reactions to a food extract cause a hive at the injection site, usually within one to two minutes, and the size of the hive is measured. The site is checked and measured again after ten to fifteen minutes and compared to the saline or histamine test site. Occasionally, scratching the skin can cause a reaction called dermographism, which is swelling at the scratch site. It is important that the allergist is informed if this type of reaction occurs normally when scratched so results are not confused with an allergen reaction. A positive reaction indicates the presence of IgE antibodies to the test food and only *suggests* that there may be an allergy. Negative results are usually more reliable than positive results and false positives occur 50–60 percent of the time. Although neither skin nor blood tests definitely confirm a food allergy, they are a fairly reliable indicator of what may be causing symptoms. Further testing is still necessary after blood and skin tests.

If RAST or skin prick tests are strongly positive or inconclusive, a trial elimination diet is tried. Elimination diets remove specific foods and/or ingredients from the diet over a two- to four-week time period. This diet, while difficult to follow at times, must be strictly followed for accurate results. If symptoms improve significantly, a diagnosis of a food allergy may be made. However, most allergists initiate a food challenge at the end of this time period. During the food challenge, eliminated foods are reintroduced into the diet one at a time. Any symptoms that occur are recorded for each individual food reintroduced. Results from both the elimination diet and the food challenge, along with RAST scores, skin tests, a detailed medical history, record of symptoms, and physical exam are used to make a firm diagnosis. Occasionally, the food will be eliminated again to confirm the diagnosis and remove all doubt.

A double-blind, placebo-controlled food challenge (DBPCFC), although not routinely performed by allergists, may be used to confirm results from the elimination diet. Long considered the gold standard of allergy testing because results are extremely accurate, it also has a high potential to cause severe allergic reactions. Therefore, it should only be performed under strict medical supervision and with access to emergency medical services. During this test, a "safe food" that has been injected with a specific amount of the suspected allergen is eaten, and then a "safe food" that has no allergens in it is eaten. This is done to "blind" the individual so that true reactions can be distinguished from pseudoallergic reactions, thus ensuring objective results. The individual is observed over a period of time for any reactions. As long as there are no reactions, doses of the

Table 2.5
Sample Elimination Diets

An elimination diet removes allergenic foods from the diet for a two- to four-week time period. Two approaches can be taken: eliminating only a specific food or food group that is suspected of causing an adverse reaction based on symptoms OR eliminating every food that could possibly cause an adverse reaction. Eliminating all allergenic foods is reserved only for those who experience severe symptoms or have difficulty identifying problem foods through testing and the use of a regular elimination diet. It should *only* be followed for seven to ten days because it is extremely difficult to comply with and very limited nutritionally.

The following sample elimination diet* provides a well-balanced, nutritionally complete sample menu that can be followed for a two- to four-week time period.

Breakfast
$^1/_2$ cup apple juice
1 cup puffed corn or cream of rice cereal
1 cup enriched rice milk
1 oz. sliced grilled ham
1 tsp. unsalted, milk and soy free margarine

Lunch
3 ounces sliced grilled chicken breast
2 slices egg, milk, soy, and wheat-free bread
2 tsps. unsalted, milk and soy free margarine
1 tossed green salad with oil and vinegar dressing
$^1/_2$ cup canned pears
1 cup enriched rice milk

Supper
3 ounces roast pork
$^1/_2$ cup sweet potatoes, mashed
$^1/_2$ cup cooked broccoli
$^1/_2$ cup cooked carrots
2 tsp. unsalted, milk and soy free margarine
$^1/_2$ cup fresh pineapple
1 cup enriched rice milk

Snack
$^1/_2$ cup grapes

A strict elimination diet eliminates the eight major food allergens—egg, fish, milk, peanuts, shellfish, soy, tree nuts, and wheat—from the diet. It does *not* remove some of the more rare food allergens (i.e., corn or rice) or account for food additive hypersensitivities or food intolerances (i.e., fructose intolerance, etc).

Table 2.5 (*continued*)

___

A strict elimination diet follows these rules:
Allowed Foods
Beverages: distilled water, pear or cranberry juice*
Condiments: non-iodized sea salt
Desserts: pudding made from tapioca or rice, sweetened with pear or cranberry juice (none made with milk or eggs)
Fruits: pears, cranberries
Grains: millet, rice, tapioca
Protein: dried lentils**, rinsed well and boiled
Oils: canola, sunflower (cold pressed)
Vegetables: lettuce, parsnips, squash, sweet potatoes, yams

- All foods must be washed and cooked with distilled water only.
- Glass, iron, or aluminum cookware and utensils should be used only.
- Avoid stainless steel, plastic, and nonstick-coated cookware and utensils.
- Discuss medications that should be avoided with physician.

___

This menu provides approximately 1800 calories; increasing or decreasing portion sizes will tailor this sample menu to individual caloric needs.

*Should *only* be followed for seven to ten days; used only for those who experience severe symptoms or have difficulty identifying problem foods through testing and the use of a regular elimination diet.

**High in fructose and must be eliminated if testing for fructose intolerance or malabsorption.
Adapted from: *The American Dietetic Association Food Allergies* and Food Allergy Survival Guide.

allergen are increased until a reaction occurs, when the test is stopped. The allergist is then notified of the results. Open challenges, in which an undisguised allergenic food is eaten, may also be used as final confirmation of a negative DBPCFC test or to confirm a positive RAST or skin test.

DUBIOUS TESTING METHODS

There are a number of other tests available that claim to diagnose food allergies. Many are unproven, experimental, and very controversial. Catatonic testing (Bryan's tests) combines blood with a specific food protein and then analyzes it for the presence of white blood cells. If the numbers of white blood cells decrease, then it "diagnoses" a food allergy. Research studies have yet to prove the validity of this test and it is not regarded as accurate.

Sublingual testing or provocation-neutralization therapy requires placing a drop of a specific food protein solution under the tongue. If a reaction occurs, a second weaker solution of the same food protein is placed under the tongue and called a neutralizing dose. It is then recommended that the neutralizing dose be taken before eating the allergenic food to prevent symptoms. No research study has confirmed the effectiveness of this technique as a test or treatment, and it has the potential to produce life-threatening severe reactions.

Intradermal skin testing injects a specific food protein solution under the skin. Similar to skin prick testing, this method uses a larger needle to inject the food protein directly into the skin, increasing the risk for a serious allergic reaction. The skin is then examined for hives and reddening (erythema). False positives are common and, because of the high risk, it is not recommended.

Subcutaneous testing is similar to sublingual testing and specific amounts of food extracts are injected. If an individual has a reaction, then a more dilute solution of the food extract is injected as a neutralizing dose and treatment. Diluted food extract is then given in the form of drops to place under the tongue before eating the allergenic food. This test and treatment is very risky and unproven.

IgG testing analyzes a blood sample for the presence of food-specific IgG antibodies. Although IgG antibodies are found in both allergic and nonallergic individuals, experts think their production is a normal response to digestion. Therefore, this test is not a proven or currently recommended method for diagnosing food allergy.

Atopy patch test places a food allergen directly on the skin, which is then covered with a patch for forty-eight hours. The skin is monitored for two to three days for signs of a rash, much like that seen with contact dermatitis or poison ivy. This test can sometimes provide accurate results for delayed allergic reactions, but response is varied and still not very reliable.

In vitro assay for lymphocyte and eosinophil activation and total serum IgE screening are blood tests that measure the activity of immune cells and IgE antibodies. Neither are proven or reliable testing methods.

Food intolerance testing is offered by some labs and is becoming increasingly popular. Most are not proven methods, but the mediator release test (MRT) claims it is an accurate indicator of food sensitivities (not allergies). MRT measures the cumulative number of immune cells in the blood after exposure to specific foods or chemicals. The reaction is then categorized as reactive, moderately reactive, or nonreactive. One European study found MRT was quite accurate in identifying milk sensitivity in children (Melina, 2004). However, no other studies have validated the accuracy of the MRT, and it is still considered an unproven and experimental method.

Various other testing methods that use muscle strength, hair and blood samples that analyze the effect foods have on cells, and skin electrical resistance have yet to be proven and some defy logic. Take the case of eleven-old-month Andrew, who had severe atopic dermatitis (Sicherer, 2006). Prior to seeing a medical allergist, Andrew's mother had him "tested" for food allergies by using the muscle strength test. In this test Andrew's mother was instructed to hold Andrew and also hold a jar of Andrew's infant baby food or formula. If the food she was holding caused her strength to lessen, Andrew was then allergic to it. But if he could tolerate the food, her strength remained consistent. As can be seen in just this one example, questionable testing methods may actually be risky and delay appropriate treatment options, while also taking advantage of those who are vulnerable.

3

Who's at Risk?

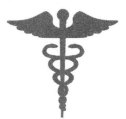

I s it possible to prevent food allergies? This is one question many parents of children with food allergies think about. In 2000 the American Academy of Pediatrics (AAP) issued guidelines for parents with a family history of allergies. These guidelines recommended that the introduction of solid foods, especially allergenic foods, should be avoided until infants were at least six months of age or older. The AAP also recommended that cow's milk should not be introduced into the diet until after the age of one, eggs after the age of two, and fish, peanuts, and tree nuts after the age of three. Pregnant and lactating women were advised to avoid eating allergenic foods, especially peanuts. These recommendations advocated avoiding exposures to known allergenic proteins in the diet until an infant's gastrointestinal tract was mature enough to appropriately handle potential food allergens. Thus, the mature gastrointestinal tract would be better equipped to digest and eliminate them while possibly preventing or delaying the onset of food allergies and hypersensitivities. But studies have yet to show that these avoidance diets work, and some are beginning to reveal that delayed introduction of food allergens may actually increase the chances of developing a food allergy. Numerous theories have been put forth about why allergies occur and these theories and research efforts will be examined in this chapter.

GENETICS, ENVIRONMENT, OR SOMETHING ELSE?

We know food allergies and hypersensitivities tend to occur in families. Identical twins have a 64 percent chance of sharing a peanut allergy, whereas nonidentical twins have only a 7 percent chance (Sicherer, 2000). While this research confirms a strong genetic link for peanut allergies, children in the same family don't always share the same allergy and risk decreases for each sibling subsequently born. This fact leads to the indisputable assumption that more than genetics are involved. There are many theories about why allergies develop in the first place and why they appear to be on the rise worldwide. Some studies point to the fact that the human immune system is increasingly attacking harmless proteins because it has less work to do and is "bored." But why this happens remains unclear. One study links allergies to geography, finding Americans who live in the South are less susceptible to anaphylaxis and those living in eastern states have higher allergy rates than those living in western states (Camargo, 2007). At this time only theories provide possible answers. Researchers suspect the following factors influence food allergy susceptibility.

- Genetics
- The hygiene hypothesis
- Age and intestinal tract immaturity
- "Leaky gut" hypothesis
- Environmental exposures
- Agricultural methods and increased reliance on processed foods

Genetic factors appear to have the strongest influence on food allergy and hypersensitivity susceptibility. Allergies "run" in families. If both parents have allergies, their children have a 70–80 percent chance of developing allergies (although not necessarily the same one). If only one parent has an allergy, this risk drops to 40–50 percent (Sicherer, 2006). If neither parent has an allergy, the child's risk drops even lower to 10–15 percent (ACAII, 2008, http://www.acaai.org/public/advice/foods.htm). Thus, all allergies, including food, are inherited to a certain extent. But genetics doesn't account for allergic individuals who have no family history of allergies. Other factors also appear to influence the prevalence of food allergies and hypersensitivities.

The hygiene hypothesis is one popular theory that suggests living in developed nations, where cleanliness is an obsession and parasitic diseases are rare, ultimately creates an increased susceptibility to allergens. Frequent use of antibacterial soaps and cleaning products, the overuse of antibiotics for human and animal illnesses, few parasitic diseases, and vaccinations that eradicate many deadly diseases are thought to decrease germ exposure as well as immunity. This in turn forces an idle immune system to look for something to do by fighting harmless food and airborne allergens instead. A 2005 report in *Nature News* highlighted the important role parasites play in asthma and allergy incidence (Schubert, 2005, http://www.nature.com). This theory is also linked to the increased number of autoimmune diseases (arthritis, diabetes, ulcerative colitis, etc.) diagnosed in recent years (Qin, 2007). As a result, studies using harmless parasitic worms to treat Crohn's disease and colitis are currently being investigated (Wilson, 2005).

Other recent studies are linking a "too clean environment" as a contributing factor for inflammatory bowel diseases (Klement, 2008). Some of these studies show that children who attend day care, grow up on farms, live with pets, or are born later in the family order have decreased rates of allergies and asthma. Yet, those who live in the inner city have some of the highest rates of asthma, suggesting that factors other than hygiene are also involved. (Science Daily, 2006, http://www.sciencedaily.com).

Age and intestinal immaturity are also thought to have some influence on allergy susceptibility. At least 80 percent of food allergies develop by the age of one (Wood, 2007). The digestive system of an infant is immature until six months of age. This immature gastrointestinal tract does not provide a developed protective barrier against allergenic proteins, thus allowing them to cross into the bloodstream and sensitize a child to a particular food. Although rare, sensitization has occurred in utero, when allergenic proteins in the mother's diet cross the placenta and subsequently sensitize the unborn baby to them. Some research indicates that the timing of the first exposure to an allergen may contribute to food allergy onset. This happens in one of two ways: either through continuous low-dose exposures at a young age or via large-dose exposures that occur periodically during childhood. Repeated low-level exposures early in life happen during breast-feeding, when first introducing solid foods, or via inhalation, and may possibly sensitize a child to that specific allergen. Large-dose exposures early in life may exceed an individual's "threshold" tolerance level, thus exceeding the amount they can tolerate without symptoms and triggering an allergic response.

Food allergies often worsen during the first two to three years of life, when the gastrointestinal tract is mature. Thus, the validity of this theory remains questionable. Concerns about maternal diet and the immature gastrointestinal system of the infant prompted the AAP to issue eating guidelines for infants in 2000. However, review of study results since that time prompted the AAP to revise these guidelines and reissue new ones in January 2008. These new guidelines recommend infants born into high-risk families be breast-fed for at least four months (preferably one year) and the introduction of solid foods be delayed until four to six months of age. If breast-feeding is not feasible, then the use of hypoallergenic (hydrolyzed) infant formulas (*not* soy based) is recommended. Previous recommendations for women to avoid eating peanuts during pregnancy and breast-feeding have not been found to decrease allergy risk, and these recommendations were eliminated for mothers (Greer, 2008), although one recent study did indicate daily consumption of peanuts in the maternal diet increased asthma risk for unborn children (Willers, 2008). Although this one study still needs to be validated by others, it has been shown by other studies that avoidance diets may actually increase food allergy risk in mice (although the implications for humans remain unknown) (Sicherer, 2006).

Although infants and children are at the highest risk for developing allergies, they also have a greater tendency to outgrow them. Approximately 90 percent of children allergic to soy and wheat outgrow these allergies by their third birthday. Around 85 percent outgrow allergies to egg and cow's milk by their fifth birthday (Sicherer, 2006). However, two recent studies find the length of time to outgrow an allergy is changing, and it may actually take longer than originally thought to outgrow a food allergy, if ever. These studies, reported in the *Journal of Allergy and Clinical Immunology*, found 4 percent of children with an egg allergy outgrew it by age four, 12 percent by age six, 37 percent by age ten, and 68 percent by age sixteen (Savage, 2007). Of those with milk allergy, 19 percent outgrew it by age four, 42 percent by age eight, 64 percent by age twelve, and 79 percent by age sixteen (Skripak, 2007). Allergies to fish, peanuts, shellfish, tree nuts, or some fruits and vegetables and those with food hypersensitivities, such as lactose intolerance, rarely resolve because most develop over time.

The leaky gut hypothesis speculates that "leaky gut" syndrome, also known as increased intestinal permeability, is to blame for food allergies. An unhealthy gastrointestinal tract is thought to make the intestinal lining more permeable, allowing allergens to pass through into the bloodstream, which then sensitizes the individual to that allergen and triggers an immune response. Increased permeability may be caused by inflammation, injury to the intestinal wall, injury to the normal bacteria that live in the intestines, and stress. Diseases, such as Crohn's and ulcerative colitis, inflame the intestinal wall. Chemotherapy drugs or radiation treatments to the abdomen used in cancer treatments, excess alcohol consumption, nonsteroidal anti-inflammatory drugs (NSAIDs), and stress may also damage the intestinal lining. Antibiotic drugs may destroy good bacteria that normally reside in the intestine, allowing unfriendly bacteria to flourish and cause problems. Diet choices, such as diets high in sugar, may have a negative effect on the "good" intestinal bacteria present in the gut. The existence of leaky gut syndrome remains very controversial, one that many gastrointestinal physicians do not support. However, one recent study showed rogue enzymes in the body may damage intestinal lining (Delano, 2008, online *Hypertension*), causing a leaky gut as well as diabetes and hypertension. Other studies are finding the use of probiotics in the diet improves gastrointestinal health and may prevent allergies in infants (Furrie, 2005).

Environmental exposures include use of antacids, food additives, vaccines, vitamins, and exposure to tobacco smoke or other environmental toxins. A 2004 study, reported in *Pediatrics*, found dietary vitamins could distort T cell activity and actually participate in inflammatory and allergy responses. This study found early vitamin supplement use in exclusively formula-fed children increased risk for food allergies (Milner, 2004). Antacids, which suppress stomach acids, are thought to reduce the ability to break down allergenic proteins in the stomach, making them more potent. Vaccinations are thought to decrease the workload of the immune system and, therefore, increase allergen susceptibility because the immune system is "looking" for something to do. There has been a strong association between tobacco smoke exposures in infancy and a stimulated immune system resulting in allergies, in particular asthma (Barclay, 2007, online Medscape Medical News). Other environmental pollutants may also have the same effect as tobacco, although studies have yet to make any strong connections. No clear evidence yet links food allergies with antacid use. Neither do studies prove vaccinations increase allergy risks, with the benefits of vaccinations far outweighing any associated risks.

Agricultural methods and increased reliance on processed foods may increase food allergies and adverse food reactions. Changes in our food supply over the last century have contributed to how food is procured and processed. For many years humans relied on gathering wild plants and hunting to survive. But as climates changed and glaciers melted, leaving rich, fertile soils behind, farming villages evolved. Early farmers learned which wild plants were fit for human consumption and saved their seeds to replant and harvest each year. Herds of goats, sheep, and other useful animals were captured and bred for their useful traits and for milk production. Humans gradually transitioned from a hunting and gathering society to an agrarian society dependent on food production methods. During the 1800s in America, the Industrial Revolution changed the economic landscape. Mills and factories expanded and waterways and railroads were built to ship goods long distances. Farm equipment and food processing and packaging inventions made farming easier, food distribution faster, and exports to other regions and countries possible. Other developing nations followed along this same path.

Today, consumers in Westernized countries are increasingly dependent on supermarkets for the staples of their diet. Increasing numbers of meals are ready-made or eaten in restaurants. But ease of food accessibility comes with a price. Frequent use of preservatives is required to increase food shelf life and prevent growth of dangerous bacteria. Mass-produced meat and produce require the use of pesticides and antibiotics. Pesticides and herbicides, substances intentionally designed to destroy insects and increase crop yields, and antibiotic use in meats, used to keep animals healthy and increase yield, have been blamed for adverse food reactions among other things. In addition, increased food imports from other regions or countries increase exposures to food allergens not indigenous to the culture, thereby introducing new food allergens to a population that may be susceptible to them.

Active research into crop modifications that reduce food allergens is currently underway. While removing food allergens from a food may allow some allergic individuals to eat foods they cannot eat now, genetic manipulation of foods also has a dark side. Genetic modifications of crops, used mainly to increase crop yields and improve disease and insect resistance, has the potential to introduce new allergens into foods previously assumed to be "safe." The Food and Agriculture Organization of the United Nations (FAO) and World Health Organization (WHO) issued a report about foods derived from biotechnology in 2000 that concluded, "... the gene product should be assumed to be allergenic unless proven otherwise. The transfer of genes from commonly allergenic foods should be discouraged unless it can be documented that the gene transferred does not code for an allergen" (FAO/WHO, 2000). The WHO/FAO report recommended, although their recommendations are not binding, that all genetically modified foods should undergo safety assessments, including analysis of nutritional aspects and relationship to medical disorders, before being introduced into the food supply for human consumption.

StarLink corn, a genetically modified grain in the United States, is one example of the potential dangers of exposing consumers unknowingly to new food allergens in foods where they do not naturally occur. A specific protein was genetically added to the corn molecule to form StarLink corn. This genetic modification allowed the corn molecule to incorporate a natural pesticide into its structure. Originally intended for use in animal feed only, this modified corn was accidentally introduced into the human food supply. Mainly used to make taco shells, some individuals with no previous history of corn allergy experienced anaphylactic reactions. Eventually, this life-threatening reaction was traced back to the genetically added protein in the StarLink corn. Subsequently, StarLink corn was banned from the market. However, as of 2003, approximately 1 percent of U.S. corn crops were reported to still be contaminated (Melina, 2004).

StarLink corn is not the only genetically modified crop that has caused problems. Soy plants were genetically engineered with chemical toxins in 1996 to increase crop profits. This genetic modification created a new soy protein 41 percent identical to the peanut allergenic protein Ara h 3. Within five years, from 1997 to 2002, peanut allergies doubled after the introduction of this new soy protein into the food supply (online AllergyKids.com). As a result, the British Dietetic Association advises parents to delay introduction of soy into the diet until after age one. In France, parents are advised to delay the introduction of soy into the diet until after age three.

Genetics, reaching a "threshold" amount of allergen tolerance beyond which an allergy or hypersensitivity develops, decreasing amounts of digestive enzymes, sensitivities to food additives, or cross-reactivity reactions are all thought to influence the development of a food allergy or hypersensitivity. Regardless of these theories, which are all credible, most experts agree that family history still remains the best predictor of food allergy or hypersensitivity susceptibility at this time.

RESEARCH EFFORTS

It must be kept in mind when evaluating scientific studies that not all studies are well designed or include a large enough sample of study participants to be applicable to the general population. The guidelines outlined by the United States FDA (available on the USFDA Web site under "Evidence-Based Review System for the Scientific Evaluation of Health Claims," http://www.cfsan.fda.gov/~dms/hclmgui5.html#intro) are useful when evaluating the validity of scientific study results. In general, when looking at a study, always consider the following:

- What scientific rationale was used? Did the study specify and measure the substance that is the subject of the claim?
- What type of study design was used—animal or in vitro, cohort, case-control, cross-sectional, intervention, observational, research synthesis? Was the study double-blind, placebo–controlled, or random?
- Did the study appropriately specify and measure the disease or health-related condition that is the subject of the claim? Were extraneous factors controlled and measurement standards appropriate and relevant?

- What end points were used? Was the study relevant to the human population? How many study subjects participated? Were outcomes consistent?
- Were conclusions based on findings? Was appropriate statistical analysis used? Were results relevant when applied to practical situations?
- Were results published in a peer-reviewed journal? Have findings been reproduced by other researchers?

As seen in a previous chapter, food allergies and hypersensitivities appear to be increasing worldwide. In the United States, the National Institutes of Health (NIH) was given authority by the Food Allergen and Consumer Protection Act of 2004 to enhance and coordinate food allergy research activities. In 2005 the European Union initiated the multidisciplinary project EuroPrevall to study food allergies and develop diagnostic tools and databases. In addition, many private and philanthropic organizations and advocacy groups sponsor and fund food allergy research. Attention to factors that trigger food allergies and improve methods of detection and treatment has never been greater. Government agency commitment to provide economic incentives and funding are beginning to draw researchers to this important research area.

As a result, preliminary research studies are beginning to identify lipid and lipid-carbohydrate complexes that appear to trigger immune and allergy responses. A special type of T cell, called a natural killer T (NKT) cell, has been identified that appears to be involved with asthma and food allergies in mice. X-ray crystallography and nuclear magnetic resonance imaging can now identify three-dimensional protein structures and protein-protein interactions, allowing a better understanding of food allergens and IgE antibodies that can lead to new treatments. Advances in the Human Genome Project, a collaboration between the U.S. Department of Energy and the NIH, which is working to identify the gene components of DNA, and the International HapMap Project, a multicountry endeavor to identify and list genetic similarities and differences, create opportunities to identify the genetics of food allergens.

Research areas evaluating new prevention and treatment methods are promising as studies look at the mucosal introduction of food allergens, rush immunotherapy (a type of immunotherapy that rapidly increases dose levels of an allergen over a period of time), probiotics, and early life, high-dose allergen exposures. Of course, researchers still face challenges as well. Clinical allergy studies applicable to people are inherently risky. Government funding agencies may not recognize the merit of a proposed study and deny funding. Legal permission of parents or guardians is required when studies involve infants or children. Humane treatment of animals must be overseen in lab animal studies. Funding may necessitate pharmaceutical company associations. The cause and effect of study results may not always be apparent at the end of the study.

The NIH Expert Panel on Food Allergy Research (a collaboration between the NIH and National Institute of Allergy and Infectious Diseases [NIAID]) convened in March 2006 and recommended five research areas that efforts should be focused on to ensure progress in food allergy research (NIH and NIAID, 2006, http://www3.niaid.nih.gov). These recommendations included improvements and advances in: (1) clinical trial design, (2) clinical trials to prevent and treat food allergy, (3) epidemiology and genetics of food allergy, (4) basic and preclinical research studies, and (5) research resources.

SELECT CLINICAL STUDIES

The following section provides a short list of relevant food allergy and hypersensitivity studies. More may be found in the bibliography. When looking at these studies, remember to keep in mind research evaluation guidelines when assessing their results. Most government agencies and food allergy organizations post research updates periodically and are worth perusing to remain up-to-date on the latest findings.

Food Allergies

Allen, L. 2008. "Priority Areas for Research on the Intake, Composition, and Health Effects of Tree Nuts and Peanuts." *The Journal of Nutrition* 138: 1763S–1765S.

Arnold, DM, Blajchman M, DiTomasso J, et al. April 23, 2007. "Passive Transfer of Peanut Hypersensitivity by Fresh Frozen Plasma." *Archives of Internal Medicine* 167(8): 853–854.

Burks, AW. May 3, 2008. "Peanut Allergy." *The Lancet* 371: 1538–1546.

Davis PA, Jenab M, Vanden Heuvel JP, et al. 2008. "Tree Nut and Peanut Consumption in Relation to Chronic and Metabolic Diseases Including Allergy." *The Journal of Nutrition* 138: 1757S–1762S.

Fernández-Rivas, M, Bolhaar S, González-Mancebo E, et al. August 2006. "Apple Allergy across Europe: How Allergen Sensitization Profiles Determine the Clinical Expression of Allergies to Plant Foods." *The Journal of Allergy and Clinical Immunology* 118 (2): 481–488.

Institute of Food Research. July 3, 2007. "Allergy Molecule Identified". *ScienceDaily*, http://www.sciencedaily.com/releases/2007/07/070702084242.htm.

Jenkins, J, Breiteneder H, Mills, C. December 2007. "Evolutionary Distance from Human Homologs Reflects Allergenicity of Animal Food Proteins." *The Journal of Allergy and Clinical Immunology* 120 (6): 1399–1405.

Kummelinga, I., Thijs, C., Huber, M., et al. 2008. "Consumption of Organic Foods and Risk of Atopic Disease during the First Two Years of Life in the Netherlands." *British Journal of Nutrition* 99: 598–605.

Lack, G., Fox, D., Northstone, K., et al. March 13, 2003. "Factors Associated with the Development of Peanut Allergy in Childhood." *The New England Journal of Medicine* 348(11): 977–985.

Longo, G., Barbi, E., Berti, I., et al. February 2008. "Specific Oral Tolerance Induction in Children with Very Severe Cow's Milk-Induced Reactions." *The Journal of Allergy and Clinical Immunology* 121 (2): 343–347.

Mine, Y., and Yang, M. June 2008. "Recent Advances in the Understanding of Egg Allergens: Basic, Industrial, and Clinical Perspectives." *Journal of Agricultural and Food Chemistry* 56 (13): 4874–4900.

Nucera, E., Schiavino, D., Buonomo, A., et al. 2008. "Sublingual-Oral Rush Desensitization to Mixed Cow and Sheep Milk: A Case Report." *Journal of Investigational Allergology and Clinical Immunology* 18(3): 219–222.

Pereira, B., Venter, C., Grundy, J., et al. 2005. "Prevalence of Sensitization to Food Allergens, Reported Adverse Reaction to Foods, Food Avoidance, and Food Hypersensitivity among Teenagers." *The Journal of Allergy and Clinical Immunology* 116: 884–892.

Schmidt, D.A., and Maleki, S.J. 2004. "Comparing the Effects of Boiling, Frying and Roasting on the Allergenicity of Peanuts." *The Journal of Allergy and Clinical Immunology* 113: S155.

Singh, M.B., and Bhalla, P.L. June 2008. "Genetic Engineering for Removing Food Allergens from Plants." *Trends in Plant Science* 13 (6): 257–260.

Temblay, J.N., Bertelli, E., Argues, J.L., Regoli, M., and Nicoletti, C. 2007. "Production of IL-12 by Peyer's Patch-Dendritic Cells Is Critical for the Resistance to Food Allergy." *The Journal of Allergy and Clinical Immunology* 120 (3): 659–65.

Vadas, P., Gold, M., and Perelman, B., et al. January 3, 2008. "Platelet-Activating Factor, PAF Acetylhydrolase, and Severe Anaphylaxis." *The New England Journal of Medicine* 358 (1): 28–35.

Celiac and Crohn's Disease and Gluten Intolerance

Akobeng, A.K., and Thomas, A.G. 2008. "Systematic Review: Tolerable Amount of Gluten for People With Coeliac Disease." *Alimentary Pharmacology and Therapeutics* 27: 1044–1052.

Klement, E., Lysy, J., Hoshen, M., et al. July 2008. "Childhood Hygiene Is Associated with the Risk for Inflammatory Bowel Disease: A Population-Based Study." *The American Journal of Gastroenterology* 103 (7): 1775.

Lammers, K.M., Lu, R., Brownley, J., et al. July 2008. "Gliadin Induces an Increase in Intestinal Permeability and Zonulin Release by Binding to the Chemokine Receptor CXCR3." *Gastroenterology* 135 (1): 194–204.e3.

Inflammatory Bowel Disease

Mazmanian, S.K., Round, J.L., and Kasper, D.L. May 29, 2008. "A Microbial Symbiosis Factor Prevents Intestinal Inflammatory Disease." *Nature* 453 (7195): 620–624.

Siggers, R.H., Boye, M., Thymann, T., et al. August 2008. "Early Administration of Probiotics Alters Bacterial Colonization and Limits Diet-Induced Gut Dysfunction and Severity of Necrotizing Enterocolitis in Preterm Pigs." *Journal of Nutrition* 138: 1437–1444.

4

Managing Food Allergies in the Real World

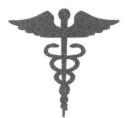

Living with a food allergy or hypersensitivity can be difficult, frustrating, and sometimes deadly. Preventing exposure to food allergens is the only way to avoid symptoms, but just avoiding an allergen is not as simple as it might seem. Many processed foods and restaurant meals contain "hidden" allergens. "Safe" foods sometimes become cross-contaminated when accidentally exposed to allergens via cooking methods, contaminated work surfaces and utensils, or during processing. Convenience foods occasionally have ingredient substitutions or changes that are not declared on the label. Food labels can be misleading; for instance, coffee creamers and margarines may be labeled nondairy, yet still contain milk proteins. Even walking through a supermarket or fish market can elicit a reaction if airborne food allergens are present and inhaled. So how can anyone with food allergies or hypersensitivities live a "normal" life? Tips and strategies to navigate the world of food will be explored in this chapter.

LIVING WITH FOOD ALLERGIES AND HYPERSENSITIVITIES

Symptoms of most Type IV hypersensitivities (nonallergic food hypersensitivities) are mostly inconvenient, disruptive, and annoying. But as a rule they are not usually life-threatening. However, "true" food allergies and some Type IV hypersensitivities (anaphylactoid reactions and some food-related medical disorders) can be deadly. Treatment of "true" food allergies and non-allergic food hypersensitivities are similar in many ways, but also different. Obtaining an accurate diagnosis from a qualified health care professional is extremely important when planning correct treatment options and living a "normal" life.

As previously discussed, any food can cause an allergic reaction. There are eight foods accountable for more than 90 percent of all food allergies world-wide. These foods are:

Cow's milk	Shellfish
Eggs	Soybeans
Fish (all species of finfish)	Tree nuts
Peanuts	Wheat

Foods naturally high in histamine content or foods and medications with food preservatives/additives that trigger histamine release from mast cells can also trigger severe reactions. The medical disorders, oral allergy syndrome, food-dependent exercise-induced anaphylaxis, and some cross-reactivity reactions are also capable of producing severe, life-threatening reactions.

Strictly avoiding a food allergen or trigger is the only proven treatment currently available. Strict vigilance of food is critical, and an effective food allergy treatment plan should always include the following components:

- Avoidance diet
- Emergency and nonemergency treatment plans
- Extra caution when eating away from home
- Label-reading skills
- Medical alert information

Avoidance diets are eating plans specifically designed to avoid the food or compound that triggers a reaction while also balancing daily nutrients necessary to maintain good health. But eating the right balance of nutrients when it is necessary to eliminate one or more food groups can be a challenge. Working with a registered dietitian is well worth the investment of time and money to ensure a nutritionally balanced and safe diet plan specifically tailored to the individual. Yet there are general diet guidelines that can be followed and these will be detailed later in this chapter.

Treatment plans save lives. In general, anyone who has experienced or has the potential to experience a severe reaction, such as anaphylaxis, will be given a prescription for an epinephrine autoinjector. This medication comes in two different strengths: junior (for children or anyone between thirty-three and sixty-six pounds) and regular (for adults or those over sixty-six pounds). The best known brands of epinephrine autoinjectors are EpiPen® Jr., Epi-Pen®, Twinjet®, and Ana Guard. Additional medications, such as antihistamines (diphenhydramine [Benadryl®]; histamine-2 receptor antagonists [H2] blockers [Zantac® or Tagamet®]); inhalant asthma medications (Albuterol); and corticosteroids (Prednisone) may also be prescribed and combined with epinephrine when symptoms are life-threatening.

Carrying the right medications at all times and in all circumstances is extremely important, even if severe reactions are rare or circumstances appear nonthreatening. A 2008 study at the University of Michigan found only 50 percent of college students with food allergies avoided eating the food they were allergic to. Twenty percent carried an epinephrine autoinjector with them at all times, and 43 percent had some other emergency medication with them at all times (University of Michigan Health System, 2008, online *Science Daily*). These study results highlight the tragic case of nineteen-year-old James, who had a peanut allergy. James ate a chocolate chip cookie at his girlfriend's house and immediately experienced itching in his mouth and throat, alerting him to the fact that a severe reaction was imminent. But he had never had a severe reaction before and had not filled his EpiPen prescription. By the time paramedics arrived to provide emergency treatment ten minutes later, his heart had stopped, and it was too late to save him (Sicherer 2006). *Life-threatening reactions can occur at any time and from foods that appear safe.* It is also important to know that not all states allow paramedics to carry epinephrine.

Besides carrying medications at all times, it is equally important to become familiar with and practice how to use a prescribed epinephrine autoinjector and educate family, friends, coworkers, and teachers about how to manage an anaphylactic emergency. The University of Michigan study also found less than half of elementary school staff recognized and knew how to respond to a food allergy emergency and less than one-third of reactions were treated with epinephrine immediately. This lifesaving treatment was often delayed for fifteen minutes or longer.

For anyone with food allergies or life-threatening hypersensitivities and their caregivers, it is critically important to recognize symptoms early, give immediate treatment with the right medications, and seek medical care quickly to minimize the chance of severe reactions such as anaphylaxis. Most fatal anaphylactic reactions follow a clear pattern. They usually involve young adults or teenagers who have asthma and peanut or tree nut allergies, who ate away from home, and who didn't carry epinephrine medications with them.

Even after symptoms appear to be under control, the individual must continue to be monitored for at least four hours for signs of delayed reactions (known as biphasic reactions). In anaphylactic reactions, both the respiratory and cardio-vascular systems are involved. Individuals with asthma and food allergies *or* a prior history of anaphylactic reactions are at high risk for severe and potentially fatal reactions. Responding to severe reactions and emergencies will be discussed in more detail in the next chapter.

Non-life-threatening symptoms do not typically involve the respiratory and/or cardiac systems and may not require an injection of ephinephrine in general, although this is not always the case. The following treatment options can help to alleviate the discomfort of less severe symptoms.

- **Skin rashes (eczema) and hives**[*]
  - Lukewarm baths or wet wraps (Aveeno® oatmeal baths can offer soothing relief) followed by liberal application of petroleum jelly or moisturizing creams (*not* lotions) to seal in moisture and prevent drying.
  - Oral over-the-counter antihistamines—Benadryl®, Zyrtec®, Clarinex®, or Allegra®—to help relieve itching. Liquid, fast-melt, or chewable forms of these medicines provide the fastest relief.
  - Over-the-counter hydrocortisone ointments are effective and safe to decrease itching. Prescription steroid ointments work but are stronger and not safe for young children.
  - Antibiotics for skin infections.
  - Avoidance of soaps, detergents, clothes, or lotions that aggravate the skin.
- **Gastrointestinal symptoms**[**]
  - Antihistamines are usually sufficient for treating abdominal pain, nausea, vomiting, and diarrhea. But worsening of symptoms must be monitored.
- **Breathing symptoms; in general all respiratory symptoms are considered life-threatening**[***]
  - Bronchodilating medications may reduce the swelling of bronchioles in the lungs and ease breathing difficulties.

---

[*]Hives can progress to life-threatening symptoms and must be monitored closely. All the above treatments will alleviate the symptoms of hives, but epinephrine may become necessary if a reaction worsens or becomes severe.

[**]If symptoms persist or worsen, an injection of epinephrine and intravenous fluids may become necessary.

[***]Ephinephrine injections or mist spray into the lungs may become necessary for severe breathing problems.

- Allergic rhinitis can be managed with nasal sprays and/or leukotriene blockers (i.e., Singulair®).
- Intravenous or oral steroids may reduce swelling in the throat and lungs.

Extra caution is always needed when living with food allergies. Unfortunately, many people do not think food allergies are a serious threat to life. Take the case of Irene, who had a severe allergy to nuts and was dining out at an Italian restaurant. Irene carefully questioned the waitress about a menu item, checking to be sure it was not made with nuts. The waitress, who unfortunately didn't take Irene's allergy seriously, assured her it did not even though she never checked with the kitchen staff. But the meal included a sauce that was nut-based and Irene suffered a reaction, later dying at the hospital. As a rule of thumb, when eating away from home, *always* ask to speak directly to whoever is preparing the meal or the manager and explain the severity of a reaction to a particular food allergen. *Don't be afraid to ask*; it can mean the difference between life and death.

Contamination of "safe" foods by "unsafe" foods, called cross-contamination, is another key concern for those living with food allergies. Food-processing equipment is often shared with different food products. If cleaning between different food batches is not thorough enough, traces of potential allergens may still remain on processing equipment, contaminating the next food product that is processed. Take the case of Stephen, who has an allergy to milk. Stephen drank an apple juice pack with his lunch. After he experienced a severe reaction, which had never occurred before, an investigation revealed that the equipment used to fill the apple juice containers in the processing facility was also used to fill milk containers. Apparently, the cleaning process between foods had accidentally left milk allergens on the equipment, thus contaminating the apple juice. But contamination can even occur in processing plants that have separate processing lines for their food products via airborne allergens. Cross-contamination can occur anywhere—in the home, in restaurants, in supermarkets, and anywhere foods are kept or served. Being aware of this potential risk and asking questions helps to decrease risk.

Fortunately, many restaurants are beginning to take food allergies more seriously and are increasingly willing to work with their patrons to ensure an allergen-free meal. The New Jersey Department of Health and Senior Services, Rutgers University, and the New Jersey Restaurant Association partnered to develop the Ask Before You Eat Program (*http://www.foodallergy.rutgers.edu*), implementing Public Law 2005, c.026 (A303 ACS 2R) that targets New Jersey residents who have food allergies. Sloane Miller, a psychotherapeutic social worker with food allergies living in New York, also developed an Internet blog to help those with food allergies dine out safely. Worry-Free Dinners (http://worryfreedinners.blogspot.com) is a Web site that provides information about restaurants and chefs who offer allergy-safe meals for members of a food allergy group in the New York City area. The Food Allergy & Anaphylaxis Network implemented a restaurant training program for the National Restaurant Association and is currently planning a food allergy training program for managers and employees. Restaurants in Sweden are receiving "allergy-free" certificates if their staff undergo a special training course that teaches them about food allergies and how to meet the needs of their patrons to help them avoid allergic reactions. But even with this increased attention to food allergies, caution is still advised when eating out.

Label reading is also extremely important. In the United States the Food Allergen Labeling and Consumer Protection Act of 2004 (FALCPA) became effective January 1, 2006. Gluten must also be listed as of August 2008. FALCPA requires the top eight food allergens (eggs, fish, milk, peanuts, shellfish, soybeans, tree nuts, and wheat) to be listed on food labels by their common name if used as a food ingredient. If cross-contamination is possible where the food is processed, the food label must list a warning about this potential danger. Prior to this law, although inclusion of all ingredients was required on the food label, loopholes in food laws allowed the "Two Percent Rule." This rule did not require ingredients to be listed in order by weight if 2 percent or less of the ingredient was added. Exemptions also allowed additives to be listed as "flavors" or "spices," putting individuals at risk for unknown food allergens. Soy, a very common ingredient added to cans of tuna fish, is one example that many consumers with soy allergies were unaware of prior to this new law.

Other countries vary in their food-labeling laws, some providing more disclosure than others. Food-labeling laws in Australia, Canada, and New Zealand require food manufacturers to list the eight major food allergens used in processed foods plus sesame seeds and sulfites. In the United Kingdom all eight major allergens plus sulfites and celery, mustard, and sesame seeds must be listed if they are over a certain concentration. But even with more strict food-labeling laws, food manufacturers sometimes change ingredients without notice or cross-contamination can occur accidentally. Therefore, it is a wise habit to periodically check product alerts and recalls. The Food Allergy and Anaphylaxis Network provides a timely Special Allergy Alert page, which can be accessed at http://www.foodallergy.org/alerts.html. Health agencies of many countries and most food manufacturers also issue food alerts when food safety is in question.

Medical alert information can mean the difference between life and death. Wearing a medical identification bracelet or necklace can be lifesaving when an exposure occurs unexpectedly. If a reaction renders an individual unable to communicate, this easily identifiable accessory can allow rapid and accurate treatment before it is too late. MedicAlert® Jewelry is available at a number of different medical identification Web sites. Allergy Cards, a business card that lists food allergies and prohibited foods, can also be carried and given to restaurant chefs and wait staff. One Web site, http://www.allergycards.com, offers them at no charge. If traveling oversees, Allergy Translation (http://www.allergytranslation.com) and Select Wisely (http://www.selectwisely.com) offer cards translated into different languages for a fee. The Food Allergy Initiative (FAI) offers free Food Allergy Restaurant Cards translated into ten different languages, and these can be accessed at their Web site under the downloads tab.

AVOIDANCE DIETS

Both food allergies and hypersensitivities require changing food habits to avoid symptoms. But eliminating a food, or groups of foods, also eliminates essential minerals, nutrients, and vitamins needed for good health. Children with food allergies are frequently found to be deficient in calcium, iron, vitamin D, vitamin E, and zinc (Sicherer, 2006). Yet young children tend to outgrow most of their food allergies and food challenges should be tried (*only* with medical supervision) periodically to determine if they have outgrown their food allergy. It is recommended that children with milk, soy, and wheat allergies receive food challenges (under strict medical supervision and with access to emergency care *only*) every one to two years. Children with egg allergy are recommended to receive a food challenge every two to three years. However, fish, nut, peanut, and shellfish allergies or adult food allergies or sensitivities rarely resolve, and food challenges are not recommended for these individuals. Some food hypersensitivity reactions can diminish if a trigger food is completely avoided for a period of time. Gradually reintroducing the trigger food in small amounts may be tried. Sometimes individuals are able to eat the food again without recurring symptoms or sometimes they can tolerate it in only small amounts. But reintroducing a prohibited food into the diet, *only* under strict medical supervision, is worth the nutritional benefits it provides when adverse reactions do not recur.

Avoiding all sources of an allergenic food and maintaining a nutritionally balanced diet is challenging and requires planning and constant vigilance. In general, every meal should include at least one serving from the following food groups, depending on specific individual calorie requirements and food allergy or hypersensitivity:

- Fruits
- Vegetables
- Protein (meat, poultry, fish, legumes, seeds, or nuts, peanut butter, eggs, cottage cheese)

- Grains
- Calcium rich milk or dairy food

The American Dietetic Association Food Allergies and *The Food Allergy Survival Guide* by Vesanto Melina, Jo Stepaniak, and Dina Aronson are reliable and helpful resources for sample daily menus and to locate allergen free ingredients, recipes, and vendors. Resources are also listed in Appendix D.

While it may seem simple to avoid a problematic food, allergenic foods and ingredients can appear under different names on food labels or be "hidden." Sometimes they are used as a substitute for other ingredients. Reading and understanding a food label ingredient list is a necessary skill, even if a food is frequently eaten without incident. Regular checks of manufacturer alerts for ingredient changes or accidental contamination is important. While a safe diet varies from person to person and depends on their specific food allergy or hypersensitivity, there are some universal guidelines that may be used to avoid potential problems. Many food allergies and hypersensitivities often share the same diet restrictions and each will be examined.

DIET GUIDELINES

When looking at ingredient lists on food labels, each allergenic food has a specific set of terms that indicate it is present in that food. Table 4.1 lists each specific food allergy and the different names or terms that can be used for that particular food allergen. In general, these ingredients should always be avoided or used with extreme caution for a particular food allergy. Because food ingredients are so numerous, it is not even possible to include all of them in this book. Therefore, it is important to remember these lists are *not* comprehensive, and *any ingredient name that is questionable or unknown must be investigated before it is eaten.*

Egg Allergy

Eggs are a good source of biotin, folacin, pantothenic acid, protein, riboflavin, selenium, and vitamin B_{12}. When living with an egg allergy, it can be difficult to avoid them because many baked foods, bagels, breads, fried food breading, marzipan and some candies, marshmallows, pastas, pretzels, and commercially prepared grain products contain eggs. Besides bakery items, egg whites may be used in baby food, bouillon or consommé, coffee, ice cream and yogurt, processed meat, root beer, salad dressing, soup base, specialty coffee, and white wine. Flu vaccines are cultured in chicken eggs, so they should never be given without the advice or supervision of a physician. Table 4.1 provides a listing of foods and ingredients that may include eggs.

Table 4.1
Allergenic Foods and Their Ingredient/Term Names
These lists are not comprehensive, so it is important to investigate any ingredient name that is questionable or unknown before consuming.

Food allergy or medical disorder	Food or ingredient name that indicates problem food is or may be present—AVOID
Corn	Acetic acid
	Alcoholic beverages (ale, beer, gin, whiskey)
	Alpha tocopherol
	Artificial flavorings
	Artificial sweeteners
	Ascorbates
	Ascorbic acid
	Astaxanthin
	Baked beans
	Bakery products (check ingredients)
	Baking powder
	Barley malt
	Biscuits
	Bleached flour
	Blended sugar (sugaridextrose)
	Bread (check ingredients)
	Brown sugar
	Calcium citrate
	Calcium fumarate
	Calcium gluconate
	Calcium lactate
	Calcium magnesium acetate (CMA)
	Calcium stearate
	Calcium stearoyl lactylate
	Candy, candied fruit
	Caramel and caramel color
	Carbonated beverages (check labels)
	Carbonmethylcellulose sodium
	Carob
	Cellulose microcrystalline
	Cellulose, methyl
	Cellulose, powdered
	Cereals (check ingredients, especially presweetened)
	Cetearyl glucoside
	Cheeses – imitation and nondairy

(continued)

Table 4.1 (*continued*)

Food allergy or medical disorder	Food or ingredient name that indicates problem food is or may be present—AVOID
Corn	Choline chloride
	Citric acid
	Citrus cloud emulsion (CCS)
	Coco glycerides (cocoglycerides)
	Condiments
	Confectioners sugar
	Cookies (check ingredients)
	Corn
	Corn alcohol, corn flour, corn gluten
	Corn chips
	Corn extract
	Cornflakes
	Corn flour
	Corn fritters
	Corn meal
	Corn oil, corn oil margarine
	Corn starch
	Corn sweetener, corn sugar
	Corn syrup, corn syrup solids
	Corn, popcorn, cornmeal
	Cornstarch, cornflour
	Crosscarmellose sodium
	Crystalline dextrose
	Crystalline fructose
	Cyclodextrin
	DATUM (a dough conditioner)
	Decyl glucoside
	Decyl polyglucose
	Dextrin
	Dextrose (also found in IV solutions)
	Dextrose anything (such as monohydrate or anhydrous)
	d-Gluconic acid
	Distilled white vinegar
	Doughnuts (check ingredients)
	Drying agent
	Erythorbic acid
	Erythritol

Table 4.1 (*continued*)

Food allergy or medical disorder	Food or ingredient name that indicates problem food is or may be present—AVOID
Corn	Ethanol
	Ethocel 20
	Ethylcellulose
	Ethylene
	Ethyl acetate
	Ethyl alcohol
	Ethyl lactate
	Ethyl maltol
	Fibersol-2
	Flavorings
	Food starch
	Frozen desserts (check ingredients)
	Fructose
	Fruit juice concentrate
	Fumaric acid
	Germ/germ meal
	Gluconate
	Gluconic acid
	Glucono delta-lactone
	Gluconolactone
	Glucosamine
	Glucose
	Glucose syrup (also found in IV solutions)
	Glutamate
	Gluten
	Gluten feed/meal
	Glycerides
	Glycerin
	Glycerol
	Golden syrup
	Graham crackers
	Gravy
	Grits
	High fructose corn syrup
	Hominy
	Honey
	Hydrolyzed corn
	Hydrolyzed corn protein

(*continued*)

Table 4.1 (continued)

Food allergy or medical disorder	Food or ingredient name that indicates problem food is or may be present—AVOID
Corn	Hydrolyzed vegetable protein
	Hydroxypropyl methylcellulose
	Hydroxypropyl methylcellulose pthalate (HPMCP)
	Iced tea, presweetened
	Inositol
	Instant coffee
	Invert syrup or sugar
	Iodized salt
	Jam, jelly
	Juice drinks
	Ketchup
	Lactate
	Lactic acid
	Lauryl glucoside
	Lecithin
	Linoleic acid
	Lysine
	Magnesium fumarate
	Maize
	Malic acid
	Malonic acid
	Malt syrup from corn (barley malt is safe)
	Malt, malt extract
	Maltitol
	Maltodextrin
	Maltol
	Maltose
	Mannitol
	Margarine
	Methyl gluceth
	Methyl glucose
	Methyl glucoside
	Methylcellulose
	Microcrystalline cellulose
	Mixes – biscuit, cake, pancake
	Modified cellulose gum
	Modified corn starch

Table 4.1 (*continued*)

Food allergy or medical disorder	Food or ingredient name that indicates problem food is or may be present—AVOID
Corn	Modified food starch
	Molasses (corn syrup may be added)
	Mono and diglyceride
	Monosodium glutamate (MSG)
	Natural flavorings
	Nondairy creamers
	Olestra/Olean (fat substitute)
	Pancake syrup
	Peanut butter (check ingredients)
	Pickles, relish, sweet
	Pie filling
	Polenta (boiled cornmeal)
	Polydextrose
	Polylactic acid (PLA)
	Polysorbates (e.g. Polysorbate 80)
	Polyvinyl acetate
	Popcorn
	Potassium citrate
	Potassium fumarate
	Potassium gluconate
	Powdered sugar
	Pregelatinized starch
	Propionic acid
	Propylene glycol
	Propylene glycol monostearate
	Pudding (check ingredients)
	Saccharin
	Salad dressing (check ingredients)
	Salt (iodized salt)
	Sauces – Asian style, BBQ, spaghetti, thickened
	Semolina (unless from wheat)
	Sherbet
	Simethicone
	Sodium carboxymethylcellulose
	Sodium citrate
	Sodium erythorbate
	Sodium fumarate
	Sodium lactate

(*continued*)

Table 4.1 (*continued*)

Food allergy or medical disorder	Food or ingredient name that indicates problem food is or may be present—AVOID
Corn	Sodium starch glycolate
	Sodium stearoyl fumarate
	Sorbate
	Sorbic acid
	Sorbitan
	Sorbitan monooleate
	Sorbitan tri-oleate
	Sorbitol
	Sorghum (not all is bad; the syrup and/or grain is often mixed with corn)
	Starch (any kind that's not specified)
	Stearic acid
	Stearoyl
	Succotash
	Sucrose
	Sugar (not identified as cane or beet)
	Syrups
	Threonine (amino acid)
	Tocopherol (vitamin E)
	Tortilla chips
	Treacle (golden syrup)
	Triethyl citrate (variant of citric acid; additive)
	Unmodified starch
	Vanilla, natural flavoring
	Vanilla, pure or extract
	Vanillin
	Vegetable anything that's not specific
	Vegetables, frozen, mixed
	Vegetable gum, oil, shortening, starch
	Vinegar, distilled white
	Vinyl acetate
	Vitamin C and Vitamin E
	Vitamins
	Waffles
	Xanthan gum (polysaccharide additive)
	Xylitol (sugar alcohol)
	Yeast
	Yogurt (check ingredients)

Table 4.1 (*continued*)

Food allergy or medical disorder	Food or ingredient name that indicates problem food is or may be present—AVOID
Corn	Zea mays (sweet corn)
	Zein (a powdered corn gluten meal)
Egg	Albumin/Albumen
	Avidin
	Baking mixes
	Baking powder made with egg white or egg albumin
	Battered fried vegetables
	Bérnaise sauce
	Beverages: coffee, root beer or wine clarified with egg
	Binder
	Bread crumbs
	Breaded meats, fish, poultry
	Broth
	Bouillon
	Caesar salad dressing
	Candy – divinity, fudge
	Chocolate candy made with cream or fondant fillings
	Chocolate sauce
	Cocomalt
	Commercially prepared breads with a glaze, cakes, cookies, cream-filled pies, donuts, meringues, muffins, pancakes, waffles, whips; prepared entrees with eggs or egg by-products
	Conalbumin
	Consommé
	Coagulant
	Cream sauces made with eggs
	Croquettes
	Custards
	Dessert powders
	Duck and quail eggs
	Egg (dried, powdered, solids, white, yolk)
	Egg drop soup or soups with egg noodles or macaroni
	Egg noodles or pastas
	Egg substitutes

(continued)

Table 4.1 (*continued*)

Food allergy or medical disorder	Food or ingredient name that indicates problem food is or may be present—AVOID
Egg	Eggnog
	Emulsifier
	French toast
	Fried foods
	Frostings or icings
	Fruit whips
	Globulin
	Hollandaise sauce
	Ice cream
	Icing
	Instant Cream of Wheat
	Instant oatmeal
	Jelly beans brushed with egg whites
	Lemon curd
	Livetin
	Lecithin
	Lipovitellin
	Lysozyme (used in Europe)
	Malted beverages
	Marshmallow candy or sauce
	Mayonnaise
	Meatballs, meatloaf
	Meringue
	Nougat
	Pancakes
	Pavlova mix
	Sandwich spreads (check ingredients)
	Soups (check ingredients)
	Tempura
	Waffles
	Wine
Fish	All species of fish
	Caesar salad
	Caviar
	Egg rolls
	Fish oils (omega-3 supplements)
	Foods containing anchovies or gelatin
	Prepared seafood meals

Table 4.1 (*continued*)

Food allergy or medical disorder	Food or ingredient name that indicates problem food is or may be present—AVOID

Fish	Roe (fish eggs)
	Surimi (imitation seafood found in
	    imitation crab cakes, crab legs,
	    lobster, lump crab meat, and
	    scallops)
	Sushi
	Tempura
	Worcestershire sauce

Milk
Lactose intolerance*
Heiner Syndrome
food protein-induced
    entercolitis or
    proctocolitis syndrome
	Artificial butter flavor
	Butter, butter fat, butter oil
	Buttermilk, buttermilk cocoa
	Casein
	Caseinates (listed
	    as ammonium, calcium, magnesium, potassium,
	    or sodium caseinate)
	Cheese
	Chocolate (check ingredients)
	Cottage cheese
	Cow's milk infant formulas
	Cream
	Cream soups
	Curds
	Custard
	Dairy
	Dijonnaise
	Dried sauces, gravy mixes
	Eggnog
	Energy bars
	Feta
	Flavorings: caramel, Bavarian or coconut cream,
	    brown sugar, butter, natural flavorings
	Florentine sauce
	General Foods International Coffees
	Ghee (a clarified butter)
	Goat's milk
	Half & half
	High protein flavor or flour
	Hot cocoa or chocolate mixes
	Hungarian sauce

(continued)

Table 4.1 (*continued*)

Food allergy or medical disorder	Food or ingredient name that indicates problem food is or may be present—AVOID

Milk
Lactose intolerance*
Heiner Syndrome
food protein-induced
    enterocolitis or
    proctocolitis syndrome
	Hydrolysates (casein, milk protein, protein, whey or whey protein hydrolysate)
	Ice Cream
	Imitation cheeses and sour cream
	Instant Potato flakes
	Kefir
	Kosher foods marked "D" or "DE" or Pareve foods
	Lactaid® milk, Lactaid® ice cream
	Lactalbumin, lactalbumin phosphate
	Lactic acid starter
	Lactoferrin
	Lactoglobulin
	Lactose
	Lactulose
	Luncheon meat, hot dogs, sausages
	Margarine
	Mashed potatoes
	Milk (derivative, powder, protein, solids, malted, condensed, evaporated, dry, whole, low-fat, non-fat, and skimmed)
	Natural flavoring
	Nisin (preservative)
	Listed as "Non-dairy"
	Nougat
	Ovaltine
	Pre-condensed vegetables and pastas
	Pudding
	Quark (a type of cheese)
	Rennet casein
	Ricotta cheese
	Sherbet
	Simplesse (fat substitute)
	Slim Fast
	Sour cream, sour cream solids
	Sour milk, sour milk solids
	Sports supplements (check ingredients)

Table 4.1 (continued)

Food allergy or medical disorder	Food or ingredient name that indicates problem food is or may be present—AVOID
	Whey (in all forms including sweet, delactosed, and protein concentrate)
	Whipped cream toppings
	Yogurt
	Yoo Hoo
Peanut	Artificial nuts (may contain other nuts)
	Asian dressings or sauces
	Baked goods (check ingredients)
	Beer nuts
	Chili
	Chinese dishes
	Chocolate (candies, candy bars)
	Cold pressed or expressed peanut oil
	Egg rolls
	Goober nuts and peas
	Ground nuts
	Hydrolyzed plant protein
	Hydrolyzed vegetable protein
	Mandalona nuts
	Marzipan
	Mixed nuts
	Nougat
	Nu-nuts™ flavored nuts (deflavored and reflavored with other nuts)
	Peanuts
	Peanut butter
	Peanut flour
	Peanut oil
	Cold-pressed peanut oil
	Peanut protein
	Soups (check ingredients)
	Thai dishes, dressings, sauces
	Satay sauce
	Vegetable oils or fats (check ingredients)
Rice	Rice
	Rice bran
	Rice flour
	Rice noodles

(continued)

Table 4.1 (*continued*)

Food allergy or medical disorder	Food or ingredient name that indicates problem food is or may be present—AVOID
	Rice starch
	Rice syrup
Sesame seed	All seeds: cotton, flax, melon, pomegranate, psyllium, pumpkin, sesame, sunflower
	Aqua Libra herbal drink
	Breads
	Bakery products
	Baked items
	Biscuits and crackers
	Chinese, Greek, Japanese, Lebanese, and Mexican dishes
	Chutney
	Confectionary items
	Energy bars
	Halvah
	Hummus
	Marinades (check ingredients)
	Mixed spices
	Muesli
	Oils: flaxseed and sesame
	Processed meats (check ingredients)
	Risotto
	Sauces (check ingredients)
	Sausages (check ingredients)
	Seasonings: celery, mustard, and poppy seeds
	Soups (check ingredients)
	Stir fries
	Tahini
	Vege burgers
Shellfish	Abalone
	Artificial crab
	Bouillabaisse
	Cerviche
	Clams
	Cockle
	Crab
	Crawfish
	Crayfish
	Fish stock

Table 4.1 (*continued*)

Food allergy or medical disorder	Food or ingredient name that indicates problem food is or may be present—AVOID
Shellfish	Lobster Mollusks Mussels Octopus Oysters Prawns Scallops Seafood flavoring Shrimp Snails/Escargot Squid

Soy
Food protein-induced
  entercolitis or
  proctocolitis syndrome
	Bouillon cubes
	Bread (check ingredients)
	Bulking agent
	Butter substitutes
	Carob
	Cereal (check ingredients), especially granola
	Chinese dishes
	Emulsifier
	Guar gum
	Ham and gerbil foods
	High energy bars
	High protein bread
	Hydrolyzed plant protein
	Hydrolyzed soy protein
	Hydrolyzed vegetable protein
	Lecithin
	Miso
	MSG
	Nato
	Natural flavoring
	Shoyu sauce
	Protein extender
	Soup (check ingredients)
	Soy (as soy albumin, flour, grits, nuts, milk, panthenol, protein, sprouts)
	Soy pasta
	Soy protein concentrate, soy protein isolate

(*continued*)

Table 4.1 (continued)

Food allergy or medical disorder	Food or ingredient name that indicates problem food is or may be present—AVOID
Soy **Food protein-induced** **entercolitis or** **proctocolitis syndrome**	Soy sauce Soybean curd, granules, oil, sprouts Sports bars Stabilizer Starch Tamari Tempeh Teriyaki sauce Texturized soy protein Texturized vegetable protein (TVP) Thickener Tofu Vegetable broth Vegetable flavorings Vegetable gum Vegetable starch Lea & Perrins® sauce Vitamin E Heinz® Worcestershire sauce
Tree nuts	Almonds, almond paste Artificial nuts Baked goods (check ingredients) Barbeque sauce Brazil nuts Breads (check ingredients) Candy (check ingredients or if cross contamination risk) Cashews Cereals (check ingredients) Chestnuts Chex mix Ethnic dishes Filberts/hazelnuts Gianduja (premium or imported chocolate mix with chopped, toasted nuts) Ground nuts Hazelnuts Hickory nuts Ice cream (check ingredients)

Table 4.1 (*continued*)

Food allergy or medical disorder	Food or ingredient name that indicates problem food is or may be present—AVOID
Tree nuts	Macadamia nuts
	Marzipan/almond paste
	Mixed nuts
	Natural extracts (artificial or imitation flavored extracts are safe)
	Nougat
	Nu-nuts™ flavored nuts (deflavored & reflavored with other nuts)
	Nut butters
	Nut extracts
	Nut flavored liquors
	Nut meal or oil
	Nut paste
	Pecans (Mashuga nuts)
	Pesto
	Pine nuts (piñon, Indian nuts, pignoli)
	Pistachios
	Pralines
	Salad dressings (check ingredients)
	Specialty cheeses or coffees (check ingredients)
	Trail mix
	Walnuts
Wheat	Baked goods (check ingredients)
	Baking powder
	Battered and breaded foods
	Bran
	Bread or bread crumbs
	Bulgur
	Candy (check ingredients)
	Cereal extract
	Corn bread
	Couscous
	Crackers and cracker meal
	Croquettes
	Dextrin
	Durum; durum flour
	Enriched flour
	Farina
	Gelatinized starch

Table 4.1 (*continued*)

Food allergy or medical disorder	Food or ingredient name that indicates problem food is or may be present—AVOID
Wheat	Gluten
	Graham flour
	Grain coffee substitutes
	Granola cereal
	Gravies
	Hydrolyzed plant and vegetable protein
	Icings
	Instant cocoa
	Kamut (ancient grain advertised as less allergenic)
	Luncheon meats
	Maltodextrin
	Matzoh
	Meatballs, meatloaf
	Modified food starch or starch
	Natural flavoring
	Pâté
	Pie crust
	Salad dressings (check ingredients)
	Sauces (check ingredients)
	Sausages
	Seasoning
	Seitan
	Semolina
	Soft wheat flour
	Soy sauce
	Spelt
	Stabilizers
	Starch
	Stuffing
	Tamari
	Tempura
	Triticale
	Vegetable gum or starch
	Vital gluten
	Wheat (bran, germ, gluten, malt, starch)
	Whole wheat berries
	Whole wheat flour

*May be able to tolerate small amounts of lactaid milk or ice cream and some dairy.

Nutrients found in eggs may also be found in legumes, meat, poultry, and whole grains. Other alternate food sources are listed in Appendices A, B, and C. Egg substitutes for use in cooking and baking can be found from specialty food companies or by checking the Food Allergy Network Web site, which offers other substitution suggestions.

Fish Allergy

In general, *all* species of fish should be avoided when an individual has a fish allergy. Fish is a good source of omega-3 fatty acids, niacin, phosphorus, protein, selenium, and vitamins B_6, B_{12}, and E. Grains, legumes, oils, and meats are also good sources for these nutrients. It remains important to read label ingredient listings of foods because some may contain fish or fish by-products. Table 4.1 contains a listing of foods and ingredients that may include fish or fish-by-products.

Cow's Milk Allergy (Lactose Intolerance, Heiner Syndrome, Food Protein-Induced Enterocolitis or Proctocolitis)

Cow's milk is found in many dairy and processed foods (butter, cheese, cream, most margarines, and yogurt). Milk is a good source of calcium, pantothenic acid, phosphorus, riboflavin, and vitamins A and D. But enriched soy, potato, or rice milks are also good sources for calcium and vitamins A and D. Nondairy calcium-rich foods are tofu made with calcium, calcium-fortified cereals, fruit juices, and some vegetables. Beans, meats, nuts, peas, peanuts, soy, and whole grains are good sources of pantothenic acid, phosphorus, and riboflavin. Alternate food sources for all nutrients found in milk are found in Appendices A, B, and C. Table 4.1 contains a listing of foods and ingredients that indicate cow's milk may be present and should be avoided by individuals with this allergy and these nonallergic hypersensitivities. The following ingredients do *not* contain milk protein and are safe to eat (even though they "sound" risky):

- Calcium lactate
- Calcium stearoyl lactylate
- Cocoa butter
- Cream of tartar
- Lactic acid
- Oleoresin
- Sodium lactate
- Sodium stearoyl lactylate

Milk is included in many processed foods, so label reading is imperative. The term "nondairy" also does *not* mean milk free. "Nondairy" coffee creamers, whipped toppings, imitation cheeses, soft-serve ice cream, and frozen desserts often contain casein or caseinates. Asian exotic fruit beverages frequently add milk. Many prescription drugs use lactose as a filler.

Lactose-intolerant individuals, infants with Heiner syndrome, and those with food protein-induced enterocolitis or proctocolitis must follow a milk-free diet as well. But some lactose-intolerant individuals can remain symptom free after eating milk and dairy products if they do not exceed a specific amount (based on individual response) of lactose or by taking lactase tablets or using Lactaid® milk or Lactaid® foods. Lactase tablets provide the missing enzyme needed to break down lactose when it is eaten, and Lactaid® milk products are sold with the lactose already broken down. However, caution is advised for any individual who has a mold or fungus allergy. A fungus is used to break down milk lactose, so Lactaid® food products and lactase tablets may trigger an allergic reaction in susceptible individuals. Anyone with a milk allergy should avoid Lactaid® milk or products because they still contain small amounts of milk protein and are, therefore, high risk.

Peanut Allergy

Peanuts are one food found in the legume family, which also includes dried beans, chickpeas, green beans, lentils, and peas. Allergies to more than one legume are rare, usually not outgrown, and are known to cause the most severe, life-threatening reactions of all the food allergies. Peanuts are a good source of chromium, magnesium, manganese, niacin, and vitamin E. These nutrients may also be found in other legumes, meat, vegetable oils, and whole grains. Listings of alternate food sources for these nutrients are found in Appendices A, B, and C. Having a peanut allergy does not necessarily mean one has a tree nut allergy.

Peanuts are added in many foods, and Table 4.1 provides a list of foods and ingredients that indicate peanuts may be present. Extreme caution should also be used with African, Chinese, and Thai dishes and some baked goods because they often contain peanuts or peanut flour.

Sesame Seed Allergy

Also known as anjoli/anjonjoli, benne seeds or oil, gingili/gingelly, oleum, *sesamum indicum*, simsim, and til or teel, sesame seeds are high in vitamin E and added to many foods. Other sources of vitamin E include almonds, broccoli, hazelnuts, kiwi, mango, peanuts and peanut butter, spinach, and corn, safflower, and wheat germ oils. Alternate food sources for sesame seed nutrients are listed in Appendices A, B, and C. Cross-contamination risks are high with all processed foods and at deli counters. Sesame may also be found in some cosmetics, some medications, and medical preparations (liniments, ointments, plasters, and soaps). Table 4.1 provides a list of foods and ingredients that indicate sesame seeds may be present.

Shellfish Allergy

Shellfish have the same nutrients found in fish. Used frequently as an ingredient in Asian dishes and stuffing, shellfish is not usually a "hidden" ingredient in foods. Kosher food products usually do not contain shellfish and are generally considered safe for anyone with a shellfish allergy (but *always* check labels before eating). Table 4.1 provides a list of foods and ingredients that indicate shellfish may be present.

Soybean Allergy (Food Protein-Induced Enterocolitis or Proctocolitis)

Soybeans are legumes and good sources of calcium, folacin, iron, magnesium, phosphorus, riboflavin, thiamin, vitamin B_6, and zinc. These nutrients are available from many other food sources (see Appendices A, B, and C), and eliminating soy from the diet is not a nutritional concern as a rule. But soy is a very common food additive in many processed foods, and eliminating it from the diet can be difficult. Table 4.1 provides a list of foods and ingredients that indicate soy may be present. Soy is commonly added to baked goods, candies and fudge, commercial ice cream and frozen desserts, energy bars, soups, canned tuna, and many other foods. Besides food, it is often found in adhesives, blankets, body lotions and creams, cosmetics, dog food, enamel paints, fabrics, fertilizers, lubricants, nitroglycerin, paper, printing inks, shampoo, and soaps. Label reading is crucial when allergic to soy. Two ingredients are exceptions: soy oil and soy lecithin. These two ingredients have had the allergenic protein removed during processing, and studies have found most people with a soy allergy, but not all, can eat them safely. Some have reported allergic reaction to them, however, so caution should be used with these ingredients.

Tree Nut Allergy

Tree nut allergies are one of the most common food allergies associated with severe anaphylactic reactions in adults. Tree nuts are good sources of monounsaturated fatty acids, copper, fiber, flavonoids, iron, manganese, magnesium, niacin, phosphorus, protein, riboflavin, selenium, thiamine, vitamin E, and zinc. Alternate food sources for these nutrients may be found in Appendices A, B, and C. Although an allergy to peanuts doesn't indicate an allergy to tree nuts, it is possible to be allergic to more than one tree nut. Tree nuts are added to many foods, and contamination risks are also very high. All food ingredients should be carefully checked before eating. Table 4.1 provides a list of foods and ingredients that indicate tree nuts may be present.

Wheat Allergy

This uncommon allergy affects an estimated one percent of infants and is usually outgrown by age three. A wheat sensitivity, however, can affect adults and is not a true allergy. Wheat is a good source of carbohydrates, chromium, fiber, iron, niacin, riboflavin, selenium, and thiamin. Alternate food sources for these nutrients are found in Appendices A, B, and C. Substitutes for wheat include amaranth, arrowroot, barley, buckwheat, corn, millet, oats, quinoa, rice, rye, and tapioca grain (although cross-contamination risks are high when these grains are processed in a facility that also processes wheat). Kamut and spelt, two ancient grains, are advertised as less allergenic. But they have been known to trigger allergic reactions and should be avoided no matter what the claim. Wheat is widely used in many foods and difficult to avoid. Table 4.1 provides a list of foods and ingredients that indicate wheat may be present.

LESS COMMON ALLERGIES

Corn allergies are rare. Like wheat, corn is difficult to avoid because it is a common ingredient in many processed foods (mostly in the form of cornstarch or corn sweeteners). Corn is a good source of chromium, iron, niacin, riboflavin, and thiamin. These nutrients may also be found in other enriched grain products and alternative food sources are listed in Appendices A, B, and C. Many commercially prepared foods, pharmaceutical items, and paper goods may have corn ingredients. Caution must be used with adhesives, baked goods, baking powder, bleached flour, breaded or fried foods, beverages, candy, canned fruits, cheese, chili, Chinese foods, cookies, gelatin capsules, jams, jellies, lunch meats, peanut butter, powdered sugar, snack foods, syrups, toothpastes, and vitamins. Some paper containers (boxes, cups, plates, milk cartons) may contain corn.

The inner surface of plastic food wrappers may also be coated with cornstarch. Safe alternatives include aspartame, baking soda, cream of tartar, fruit juices, beet or cane sugar, honey, maple syrup, potato starch, rice starch, wheat starch, and tapioca. More information about corn ingredients and foods is found at the Corn Allergens Web site, http://www.cornallergens.com/list/corn-allergen-list.php. Table 4.1 provides a list of foods and ingredients that indicate corn may be present.

Rice allergies are also rare. Rice is a good source of iron, niacin, riboflavin, and thiamin. Alternate food sources for these nutrients are listed in Appendices A, B, and C. Table 4.1 provides a list of foods and ingredients that indicate rice may be present.

LIVING WITH NONALLERGIC FOOD HYPERSENSITIVITIES

Other abnormal reactions to food—intolerances, medical disorders, and idiosyncratic reactions—may also follow the same treatment plan of appropriate medical treatment, strict avoidance diets, and vigilance. Although even an extremely small amount of a food allergen can trigger a severe reaction with a food allergy, an individual with hypersensitivities can often tolerate higher amounts of a food allergen without suffering symptoms. Treatment options for each of these includes the following recommendations.

Treatment for food additive reactions involve avoiding the additive in the diet and in any medications taken. Some food additives cause more problems than others. These troublesome food additives include BHA, BHT, MSG, salicylates, sulfites, tartrazine, and tyramine. Table 4.2 provides a list of foods and ingredients that indicate these food additives may be present.

BHA and BHT are antioxidants and used to keep fats in foods from going bad. MSG is used as a flavor enhancer in many prepared foods, restaurants, and seasonings. Listing MSG is voluntary, so caution is advised with all convenience and prepared foods and when dining out (especially with Chinese foods). Drinking alcohol at the same time as eating MSG may increase the effects of an MSG sensitivity. Salicylates are found naturally in many plant foods and thought to naturally protect plants against bacteria and fungus. They do not usually cause a problem when eaten as foods. But when they are concentrated, as in aspirin, some individuals suffer adverse reactions.

Sulfites prevent food spoilage and discoloration. They are frequently found in many beverages, foods, and medications. Individuals with asthma (especially those taking steroids) and some who have migraine headaches report being adversely affected by sulfites. Caution is advised with all dried fruits (raisins, etc.) and salad bars because sulfites are usually added to preserve or bleach the color. Sulfite-free dried fruits are available. Tartrazine is a food dye and also called yellow dye #5. It is used in many foods and medications and hypersensitivities have been reported. Label reading is very important if sensitive to this food coloring. Tyramine is a protein found naturally in foods, especially aged fermented foods. It can cause hypersensitivity reactions such as migraine headaches. Immediate medical attention is imperative, and vigilance about food safety is the only way to prevent allergic intoxications and food poisoning. Histamine is a chemical mediator that produces hypersensitivities and is found naturally in many foods. Table 4.2 provides a listing of foods that may contain histamine and should be avoided or used with caution.

Lactose, fructose, and gluten are responsible for most food intolerances. Lactose intolerance follows the same avoidance diet that individuals with a

Table 4.2
Foods and Ingredient/Terms That May Cause Hypersensitivities
These lists are not comprehensive, so it is important to investigate any ingre-dient name that is unknown or questionable before consuming.

Food additive or ingredient	Ingredient name that indicates is or may be present—AVOID
BHA/BHT	Cereals Convenience foods (check ingredients) Crackers Donuts Lard Margarine Oils Pastries Potato chips Roasted peanuts Shortening
Fructose	Artifical sweeteners: isomalt, mannitol, sorbitol, xylitol Baked goods Bread – white and wheat Cakes, cookies, crackers – wheat-based Cereal, wheat based Chicory-based coffee substitute beverages Coconut: cream and milk Confectioner's sugar Dried fruit Dried fruit bars Fortified wines: port, sherry, etc. Fresh fruits – apple, guava, honeydew melon, mango, nashi fruit (Asian pear), pear, papaya (pawpaw), quince, star fruit (carambola), watermelon Fructose Fruit juices, canned packing juice Fruit juice concentrate Fruits with high sugar content (grapes, lychee, persimmon) Fruit pastes and sauces: barbecue sauce, chutney, plum sauce, relish, sweet and sour sauce, tomato paste Fructose as an added sweetener

Table 4.2 (*continued*)

Food additive or ingredient	Ingredient name that indicates is or may be present—AVOID
Fructose	High fructose corn syrup (HFCS) – in carbonated drinks, catsup, fruit drinks, jams, jellies, pancake syrup, pickles, etc. and in liquid cough remedies and pain relievers and liquid pain medications
	Honey
	Juice drinks
	Legumes: baked beans, black-eyed peas, butter beans, chickpeas, kidney beans, lentils
	Maple syrup
	Meats cured in sugar or breaded
	Noodles, wheat
	Pasta, wheat
	Peanut butter, commercial varieties
	Soda
	Sorbitol
	Sports drinks
	Stone fruits (apricots, cherries, nectarines, peaches, plums)
	Sucrose
	Table sugar (beet and cane)
	Vegetables: artichokes, asparagus, beans, brussel sprouts, cabbage, leek, onion
	Some vinegars (pure distilled vinegar should not have fructose)
	Yoplait vanilla yogurt (natural flavoring ingredient is fructose)
	Medicines: Children's Tylenol, Advil, Benedryl, Zithromax, Amoxicillin
Gluten	Ale
	All forms of wheat – wheat bran, wheat germ, and wheat starch
	Baked beans, ready-to-eat meals with added thickeners
	Baking powder
	Barley malt
	Beer
	Bulgur
	Candy
	Chips, other snack foods with added seasonings
	Couscous

(*continued*)

Table 4.2 (*continued*)

Food additive or ingredient	Ingredient name that indicates is or may be present—AVOID
Gluten	Dried dates dusted with flour
	Flavorings
	Flour tortillas
	Flour used for breadings and coatings
	Grains:
	Barley
	Einkorn
	Emmer
	Farro
	Kamut
	Oats
	Rye
	Spelt
	Triticale
	Grain additives in teas and coffee alternatives
	Lager
	Malt vinegar
	Malted liquor
	Oatmeal
	Regular corn bread
	Seitan
	Semolina or durum wheat pasta
	Soups and broths with vegetable protein added
	Soy sauce
	Soymilk and other nondairy milks sweetened with malt
	Tempeh made with gluten-containing ingredients
	Udon noodles
	Wheat flour
	Worcestershire sauce
Histamine	Alcohol
	Benzoates
	Bologna
	Bratwurst
	Cheese
	Eggplant
	Egg whites
	Fermented or processed meats
	Kefir

Table 4.2 (*continued*)

Food additive or ingredient	Ingredient name that indicates is or may be present—AVOID
Histamine	Pepperoni
	Salami
	Sausages
	Scombroid fish
	Shellfish
	Smoked and pickled meats
	Spinach
	Strawberries
	Tofu
	Tomatoes
	Weiners
	Yogurt
MSG	Asian, Chinese, Thai dishes
	Flavoring – Accent, zest, etc.
	Glutamic acid
	Hydrolyzed plant protein
	Hydrolyzed protein
	Hydrolyzed vegetable protein
	Kombu extract
Salicylates	Flavored products: fruit, honey, and mint flavors
	All jams (except pear), jellies, and marmalades
	Almonds
	Apricots
	Blackberries
	Blackcurrant
	Blueberries
	Boysenberry
	Capsicum
	Champignon
	Cherry
	Chewing gum
	Chicory
	Commerical gravies, sauces
	Condiments
	Courgette (Zucchini squash)
	Cranberry
	Currants

(*continued*)

Table 4.2 (*continued*)

Food additive or ingredient	Ingredient name that indicates is or may be present—AVOID
Salicylates	Dates
	Endive
	Gherkins
	Grapes
	Guava
	Herbs and spices: anise seeds, cayenne, curry, dill, thyme
	Honey
	Hot peppers
	Licorice
	Loganberry
	Muesli bars
	Olives
	Oranges
	Peppermint candy, flavorings
	Pineapple
	Plum
	Prunes
	Radishes
	Raisins
	Raspberry
	Redcurrant
	Rockmelon
	Some flavorings
	Strawberries, strawberry flavorings
	Sweets
	Tangelo
	Tangerines
	Tomato
	Tomato based foods
	Tomato paste
	Toothpaste
	Water chestnuts
	White vinegar
	Worcester sauce
	Youngberry
Sulfites	Beer
	Beet sugar
	Bottled lemon juice (non-frozen)

Table 4.2 (*continued*)

Food additive or ingredient	Ingredient name that indicates is or may be present—AVOID
Sulfites	Bottled lime juice (non-frozen)
	Canned potatoes
	Coconut
	Cookies
	Crackers
	Domestic jams and jellies
	Dried fruits (excluding dark raisins and prunes)
	Dried potatoes
	Dry soup mix
	Fresh fruit salad
	Frozen pizza and pie dough
	Fruit toppings
	Gelatin
	Grape juices (white, white sparkling, pink sparkling, red sparkling)
	Grapes
	Gravies/sauces
	High fructose corn syrup
	Malt vinegar
	Maraschino cherries
	Molasses
	Pickled cocktail onions
	Potassium bisulfite
	Potassium metabisulfite
	Sauerkraut (and its juice)
	Shrimp
	Sodium bisulfite
	Sodium metabisulfite
	Sodium sulfite
	Soft drinks
	Sulfur dioxide
	Wine
	Wine vinegar
	Medications:
	Asthma
	Adrenalin chloride 1:1000 concentration
	Bronkosol
	Isuprel hydrochloride solution

(*continued*)

Table 4.2 (*continued*)

Food additive or ingredient	Ingredient name that indicates is or may be present—AVOID
Sulfites	**Topical eye drops**
	Pred-Mild
	Pred-Forte
	Sulfacetamide
	Prednisol (dexamethasone)
	Injectable medications
	Amikacin
	Betamethasone phosphate (Celestone)
	Chloropromazine (Thorazine)
	Dexamethasone phosphate (Decadron)
	Dopamine
	Epinephrine (Adrenaline, Ana-Kit, Epi-Pen)*
	Garamycin
	Gentamycin
	Isoetharine HCl
	Isoproterenol (injectable)
	Hydrocortisone (injectable)
	Lidocaine with epinephrine (Xylocaine)
	Meperidine (Demerol)
	Metarminol
	Norepinephrine (Levophed)
	Procaine (Novocaine)
	Prochloroperazine (Compazine)
	Promethazine (Phenergan)
	Solutions for total parenteral nutrition and dialysis
	Tobramycin
Tartrazine	Synthetic yellow azo dye
	May also be used with blue dyes to produce green shades in foods (like canned peas)
	Cake mixes
	Chewing gum
	Colored fizzy drinks
	Custard powder
	Fruit cordial
	Fruit squash
	Glycerin
	Honey

Table 4.2 (*continued*)

Food additive or ingredient	Ingredient name that indicates is or may be present—AVOID
Tartrazine	Ice cream
	Instant puddings
	Jam, jellies, marmalades
	Lemon
	Marzipan
	Mustard
	Sauces
	Soups
	Sweets
	Yogurt
Tyramine	Aged cheeses
	Avocado
	Banana
	Beer
	Chicken liver
	Chocolate
	Eggplant
	Fava beans
	Figs
	Gravies
	Plums
	Raspberries
	Red plums
	Sour cream
	Soy sauce
	Tomatoes
	Vinegar
	Wine (especially red)
	Yeast extract

*This medication should still be injected during an anaphylactic reaction.

milk allergy follow. Avoiding milk and dairy foods is necessary to avoid symptoms and requires constant vigilance. Some individuals are able to tolerate specific amounts of milk and dairy products and remain symptom free, whereas others cannot. See milk allergy and Table 4.1 for milk-free avoidance diet guidelines. Fructose intolerance and malabsorption necessitate excluding all foods containing fructose. Table 4.2 provides a list of foods and ingredients that indicate fructose may be present. Sorbitol, a sugar alcohol, must also be used with caution because it is converted to fructose during digestion.

Gluten intolerance, also called gluten-sensitive enteropathy, celiac disease, celiac sprue, nontropical sprue, and idiopathic steatorrhea, will be discussed in detail under gluten-sensitive enteropathy.

Treatment options for eosinophil-associated gastrointestinal disorders (EGID) require:

- Trial avoidance diets, elimination of many food allergens, and individual reintroduction of foods until specific food allergies are determined. Hypoallergenic infant formula is advised for infants.
- Steroid medications or an asthma inhaler.
- Antihistamine or antileukotriene medications.

Foods associated with food-dependent exercise-induced anaphylaxis (EIA) include celery, cheese, seafood (particularly shellfish), and wheat, although other foods have also been reported to trigger this adverse reaction. *Immediate* treatment requires ceasing all activity and rest. Antihistamines or epinephrine may be necessary when reactions are severe. Carrying an EpiPen, wearing a medical alert bracelet or necklace, and never exercising alone are necessary precautions. To avoid symptoms or anaphylaxis, the trigger food must be avoided before any exercise *or* physical activity delayed for *at least* four hours *after* eating a trigger food.

To remain symptom-free, eggs, milk, soy, or other suspected allergens must be avoided with food protein-induced enterocolitis or proctocolitis (allergic proctocolitis) syndrome. Infants require a hypoallergenic formula free of milk and soy. Breast-fed babies may be affected by their mother's diet because food allergens pass through into breast milk. Therefore, mothers who are breast-feeding must eliminate all suspected food allergens from their diet. Symptoms usually resolve within a few days, and this disorder is usually outgrown by age one.

Gluten contains the protein gliadin, which is found in barley, rye, and wheat. With gluten-sensitive enteropathy (celiac disease, celiac sprue, gluten intolerance, nontropical sprue, and idiopathic steatorrhea), gluten must be avoided in the diet because it causes chronic inflammation of the small intestine and severe damage to the intestinal mucosa (inner lining) over time, affecting nutrient absorption. To remain symptom-free, a strict gluten-free diet must be followed. Intestinal damage is reversible if gluten is consistently eliminated from the diet. The World Health Organization defines naturally gluten-free foods as having twenty parts per million (PPM) or less of gluten. Foods that are processed to become gluten-free are defined as having a maximum of 200 PPM of gluten. But it is difficult to measure the amount of gluten in food. A recent gluten threshold study indicates that 6 milligrams of gluten daily does not promote abnormalities in the gastrointestinal tract and is safely tolerated by *most* (not all) celiac patients. One slice of wheat bread has approximately 4.8 grams, or 4,800 milligrams, of gluten (Vega, 2008, http://www.medscape.com).

Diet restrictions for this medical disorder differ from wheat allergies because gluten is found in many other grains besides wheat. Table 4.2 provides a list of foods and ingredients that indicate gluten may be present. The following *gluten-free* grains are *safe* to eat, but *always* read labels because some of these may be mixed with wheat flour or processed in a facility that also processes wheat.

- Amaranth
- Buckwheat (kasha)
- Cassava (arrowroot)
- Chickpea
- Corn
- Flax
- Job's tears
- Millet
- Montina™ (Indian rice grass)
- Quinoa
- Rice (all varieties)
- Sorghum (milo)
- Tapioca
- Taro
- Teff
- Wild rice

Some gluten-sensitive individuals are able to tolerate oats, and some research shows that oat protein is digested differently from other gluten-containing grains. But oats can often become contaminated with other prohibited grains. If oats are tolerated, only "pure oats" processed in facilities that guarantee no cross-contamination should be eaten.

Gustatory flushing syndrome is not dangerous and resolves on its own without treatment. To prevent symptoms, spicy or tart foods must be avoided. See milk allergy diet guidelines for use with Heiner syndrome.

Digestive and inflammatory bowel diseases (IBD) are sometimes confused with food allergies because symptoms are frequently similar. IBDs are caused by unknown factors, but genetics, stress, and secondary food allergies or intolerances are strongly suspected. Although Crohn's disease, diverticulosis, diverticulitis, irritable bowel syndrome (IBS), and ulcerative colitis are not food allergies, they are sometimes worsened or triggered by a food sensitivity or intolerance to a food. Diverticulosis frequently improves by following a high-fiber diet (rich in fruits, beans and legumes, vegetables, and whole grains). Diverticulitis, especially when symptoms are acute, may improve on a low-residue diet (no skin, seeds, or nuts). IBS also appears to have food triggers, and following a high-fiber diet seems to improve symptoms.

Although no particular food has yet been irrefutably identified as a trigger for IBDs, some foods (although tolerance varies with the specific individual) have been associated as triggers and these are:

- Alcohol
- Caffeinated beverages (i.e., coffee, tea, some sodas)
- Carbonated beverages (i.e., soda, etc.)
- Chocolate
- Fatty foods (i.e., french fries, fried foods)
- Milk and dairy products

Remaining well nourished is a concern, because the resulting intestinal damage of IBDs can cause malnutrition. Diet planning and education with a registered dietitian is critical for individuals with these medical disorders to maintain good health and remain well nourished. Recent studies are beginning to show that using probiotics may restore healthy bacterial flora in the gastrointestinal tract, helping to alleviate symptoms.

Symptoms of oral allergy syndrome are usually minor and affect only the mouth and lips. But 7 percent of those who report symptoms experience involvement of other body systems (e.g., itching in the ears and severe stomach pains), and 1 percent have severe reactions (Sicherer, 2006). Treatment of oral allergy syndrome includes the following:

- Avoiding the food.
- Waiting it out; symptoms usually resolve within 20–30 minutes.
- Trying allergy shots for the related pollen, which may eliminate the related food allergy.
- Using antihistamine medications.

CROSS-CONTAMINATION

Even those individuals who carefully avoid food allergens and triggers may still experience a life-threatening reaction when there seems to be no trace of the food around. Consider the cases of Emily and Billy. Emily, who is allergic to fish, was eating out with friends when she experienced an allergic reaction after eating french fries. Further investigation uncovered the fact that the oil used to cook the french fries in this restaurant was also used to fry fish (Sicherer, 2006). Billy, a five-year-old with a milk allergy, was with his mother as she shopped for groceries. Stopping at the deli counter to buy ham, his mother gave him a few slices to eat as she continued shopping. But Billy began to cough and developed hives immediately after eating the ham slices, a reaction that had never occurred before. Speaking with the deli staff revealed that the deli slicer used to slice the ham was also used to slice cheese (Sicherer, 2006).

Both of these examples highlight the dangers of cross-contamination and the importance of being extra cautious when eating any food outside of the home. It is imperative to ask questions, check food labels, contact food manufacturers, and carry prescribed medications at all times to treat unexpected reactions. Avoiding the risks of cross-contamination and tips to use at home, at school, when dining out or away from home, and grocery shopping will be discussed in detail in chapter 6.

5

It's an Emergency!

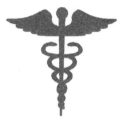

S ome foods and medical disorders can cause life-threatening reactions. Despite precautions and best efforts, accidental ingestion of food triggers can and do occur. Because there is no reliable way to predict how severe symptoms will be, anyone who has been diagnosed with a food allergy or potentially life-threatening food hypersensitivity or medical disorder should *always* be prepared for an emergency. Having an emergency plan of care helps everyone involved remain calm and focused so that rapid, lifesaving care can be given. How to handle a severe reaction and risk factors preceding them are the focus of this chapter.

TREATMENT OPTIONS

For anyone with food allergies and their caregivers, it is critically important to recognize symptoms early, give immediate self-treatment with the right medications, and seek medical care quickly to minimize the chance of a severe reaction. But there is no reliable way to predict if symptoms will remain mild or escalate into anaphylaxis. Individuals with asthma *or* a prior history of anaphylactic reactions are at high risk for a severe reaction. Their reactions should *always* be considered potentially life-threatening. But what about those who have never had an anaphylactic reaction before? How can the right treatment be given without "overreacting"?

First, anyone with a food allergy and their family, friends, colleagues, coworkers, and teachers should all be thoroughly educated about the signs of an allergic reaction and the foods that trigger them. When assessing how severe a reaction is to determine the right treatment, the following questions should be asked:

Was a trigger food eaten?
What are the current symptoms?
Are symptoms mild or severe?
Are symptoms becoming progressively worse?
How severe were past reactions?

Mild symptoms that do not worsen are rarely serious. However, if symptoms begin to involve the respiratory and cardiovascular systems (the first signs of possible life-threatening anaphylaxis) or become progressively worse, emergency care is critical and there should be *no hesitation about calling 911 and implementing a food allergy action plan, even while symptoms are still mild.* Every minute counts toward survival when a severe reaction occurs.

Two or more of the following symptoms usually indicate anaphylaxis may be imminent:

Skin symptoms (flushing, hives, swollen lips or tongue)
Difficulty breathing
Gastrointestinal symptoms (abdominal pain, vomiting)

Most fatal allergic reactions are linked to peanuts, seafood, and tree nuts (although it is possible for any food to trigger anaphylaxis). Other factors linked to fatal reactions are a confirmed diagnosis of food allergy and asthma, extreme sensitivity to a food allergen, failure to notice initial skin symptoms, and failure to receive prompt treatment with epinephrine. Teenagers and young adults are at the highest risk level for anaphylaxis because they often fail to carry emergency medications or ignore their food restrictions.

Anaphylaxis elicits an immune system response and "symptoms occur in parts of the body that have not actually contacted the food" (Sicherer, 2006). For example, if peanuts or any peanut-containing food is rubbed on the skin or eaten, a skin reaction or tingly, itchy mouth is not considered anaphylaxis because the peanut allergen came in direct contact with the affected skin area. But respiratory symptoms that become life-threatening are anaphylactic because a chemical mediator that is produced in response to the peanut allergen causes symptoms. The peanut allergen does not come into direct contact with the lungs.

Anaphylactic shock is defined as "an often severe and sometimes fatal systemic reaction in a susceptible individual upon exposure to a specific antigen after previous sensitization...." (Merriam Webster). Often individuals and family members worry that they will not recognize impending anaphylaxis. For instance, hives are often the first symptom of anaphylaxis. But many other things besides foods can cause them. Take the case of Natasha, who has an allergy to peanuts and developed a bad case of hives. Her mother called her physician to check if epinephrine should be given. A history of her symptoms revealed she had a fever and a runny nose for a few days and had not eaten any peanuts or peanut-containing foods that her mother was aware of. However, she had visited her grandmother the day before and eaten some cookies. The family physician determined that if she had eaten any peanuts accidentally, a reaction would have occurred much sooner than twenty-four hours later. Instead of giving her a shot of epinephrine, she was brought into the physician's office for evaluation (Sicherer, 2006), and her hives were diagnosed as a viral symptom. In this situation, giving an injection of epinephrine may not have been the correct treatment where hives were the only symptom. But hives *can* progress to anaphylaxis and must be closely monitored at all times. Remaining calm and assessing all factors affecting symptoms usually leads to the correct treatment option. *When in doubt, always administer emergency medications*; side effects from these medications are minor compared to reacting too slowly during a severe, life-threatening reaction.

When deciding the best way to treat an allergic reaction, the criteria outlined in Figure 1 may help to evaluate the situation objectively. In general, at the first sign of symptoms in high-risk individuals, or if symptoms appear suddenly and affect breathing or the cardiovascular system, a shot of epinephrine along with a dose of oral liquid antihistamine should be given. Emergency services (911) should be called immediately and treatment given at the nearest hospital as quickly as possible. Even when symptoms appear to be under control or over, delayed reactions (known as biphasic reactions) can still occur and the individual must be monitored for at least four to six hours after symptoms first appear.

FOOD ALLERGY ACTION PLAN

An allergy action plan is a written summary of the important treatment steps that must be followed during a reaction. Every individual who lives with a food allergy or life-threatening food hypersensitivity should carry a food allergy action plan and emergency care kit at all times. The physician or allergist will decide what medications are appropriate and help to formulate this plan for use during a reaction.

Table 5.1
Allergic Reaction Symptoms That May Become Life-Threatening

Body system	Symptoms
Respiratory	Change in voice/hoarseness
	High pitched noises when breathing
	Pale or blue skin color
	Repetitive coughing
	Shortness of breath
	Throat tightness
	Troubled breathing
	Wheezing
Gastrointestinal	Difficulty swallowing
	Swollen tongue
	Throat obstruction
Cardiovascular	Chest pain
	Dizzy or lightheaded
	Fainting
	Loss of consciousness
	Low blood pressure
	Rapid or weak pulse
Other	Feeling of doom

Table 5.2
Allergic Reaction Symptoms That Are Not Usually Life-Threatening

Body system	Symptoms
Respiratory	Occasional cough
	Nasal congestion
	Runny nose
Gastrointestinal	Abdominal pain
	Diarrhea
	Itchy mouth or ears
	Lip swelling
	Nausea
	Odd taste in mouth
	Vomiting
Skin	Eczema
	Edema
	Flushing
	Hives
	Itch
Other	Red, itchy eye
	Uterine contractions

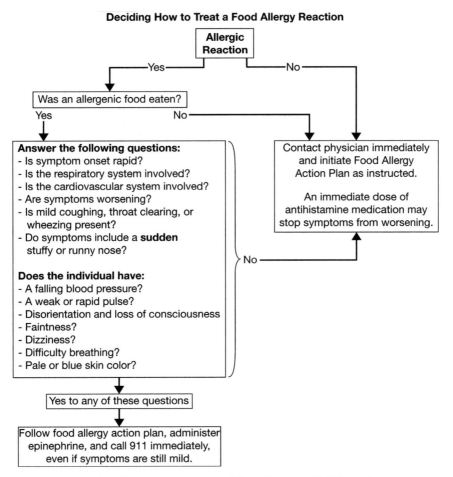

Figure 5.1. Deciding How to Treat a Food Allergy Reaction [Jeff Dixon].

A food action allergy plan should include all of the following information:

List of foods that cause an allergic reaction
List of symptoms indicating an allergic reaction
List of prescribed medications and doses
Sequence of steps to follow when treating a reaction
Names and phone numbers of three emergency contacts
Name and phone number of physician and hospital
Written statement from physician outlining this treatment plan.

(This is especially important when traveling or unable to see the regular physician. Lifesaving care may be delayed when seen by physicians who are unfamiliar with the medical history of the individual.)

Food Allergy Action Plan

Student's Name:_____ **D.O.B:**_____ **Teacher:**_____

ALLERGY TO:_____

Asthmatic Yes* ☐   No ☐   *Higher risk for severe reaction

Place Child's Picture Here

◆ STEP 1: TREATMENT ◆

Symptoms:		**Give Checked Medication**:** **(To be determined by physician authorizing treatment)	
▪	If a food allergen has been ingested, but *no symptoms*:	☐ Epinephrine	☐ Antihistamine
▪ Mouth	Itching, tingling, or swelling of lips, tongue, mouth	☐ Epinephrine	☐ Antihistamine
▪ Skin	Hives, itchy rash, swelling of the face or extremities	☐ Epinephrine	☐ Antihistamine
▪ Gut	Nausea, abdominal cramps, vomiting, diarrhea	☐ Epinephrine	☐ Antihistamine
▪ Throat†	Tightening of throat, hoarseness, hacking cough	☐ Epinephrine	☐ Antihistamine
▪ Lung†	Shortness of breath, repetitive coughing, wheezing	☐ Epinephrine	☐ Antihistamine
▪ Heart†	Weak or thready pulse, low blood pressure, fainting, pale, blueness	☐ Epinephrine	☐ Antihistamine
▪ Other†	_____	☐ Epinephrine	☐ Antihistamine
▪	If reaction is progressing (several of the above areas affected), give:	☐ Epinephrine	☐ Antihistamine

†Potentially life-threatening. The severity of symptoms can quickly change.

DOSAGE

Epinephrine: inject intramuscularly (circle one) EpiPen® EpiPen® Jr. Twinject® 0.3 mg Twinject® 0.15 mg
(see reverse side for instructions)

Antihistamine: give_____
medication/dose/route

Other: give_____
medication/dose/route

IMPORTANT: Asthma inhalers and/or antihistamines cannot be depended on to replace epinephrine in anaphylaxis.

◆ STEP 2: EMERGENCY CALLS ◆

1. Call 911 (or Rescue Squad: _____). State that an allergic reaction has been treated, and additional epinephrine may be needed.

2. Dr. _____   Phone Number: _____

3. Parent_____   Phone Number(s) _____

4. Emergency contacts:
   Name/Relationship   Phone Number(s)

a. _____   1.)_____   2.) _____

b. _____   1.)_____   2.) _____

EVEN IF PARENT/GUARDIAN CANNOT BE REACHED, DO NOT HESITATE TO MEDICATE OR TAKE CHILD TO MEDICAL FACILITY!

Parent/Guardian's Signature_____   Date_____

Doctor's Signature_____   Date_____
(Required)

Figure 5.2. Food Allergy Action Plan. [2008, the Food Allergy and Anaphylaxis Network. Used with permission.]

Besides this plan, an emergency care kit should be assembled and carried at all times. This kit includes all prescribed medications and the food action allergy plan. If the individual is a child, extra kits should be kept at school and with all caregivers. Family members, friends, coworkers, teachers, etc.,

TRAINED STAFF MEMBERS

1. _____   Room _____

2. _____   Room _____

3. _____   Room _____

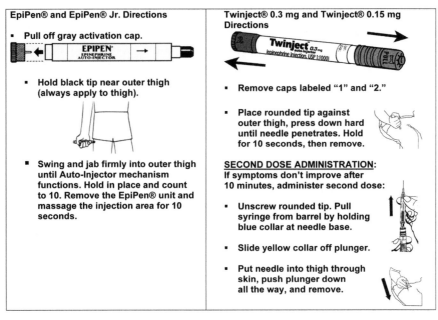

EpiPen® and EpiPen® Jr. Directions

- **Pull off gray activation cap.**

  - **Hold black tip near outer thigh (always apply to thigh).**

  - **Swing and jab firmly into outer thigh until Auto-Injector mechanism functions. Hold in place and count to 10. Remove the EpiPen® unit and massage the injection area for 10 seconds.**

Twinject® 0.3 mg and Twinject® 0.15 mg Directions

- **Remove caps labeled "1" and "2."**

- **Place rounded tip against outer thigh, press down hard until needle penetrates. Hold for 10 seconds, then remove.**

SECOND DOSE ADMINISTRATION:
If symptoms don't improve after 10 minutes, administer second dose:

- **Unscrew rounded tip. Pull syringe from barrel by holding blue collar at needle base.**

- **Slide yellow collar off plunger.**

- **Put needle into thigh through skin, push plunger down all the way, and remove.**

Once EpiPen® or Twinject® is used, call the Rescue Squad. Take the used unit with you to the Emergency Room. Plan to stay for observation at the Emergency Room for at least 4 hours.

For children with multiple food allergies, consider providing separate Action Plans for different foods.

**Medication checklist adapted from the Authorization of Emergency Treatment form developed by the Mount Sinai School of Medicine. Used with permission.

The Food Allergy & Anaphylaxis Network

June/2007

Figure 5.2. (*continued*)

should be trained in what to do during a reaction and how to give medications. EpiPen® offers an EpiPen® Trainer–Auto-Injector Training device that teaches anyone how to correctly administer emergency epinephrine (without using needles or medication). Medication expiration dates and product recalls should be checked on a regular basis and expired medications always replaced, even if rarely used. In an emergency, the money invested on replacement medications is well worth saving a life.

RISKS OF SKIN EXPOSURES, AIRBORNE ALLERGENS, AND OTHER SOURCES

Many allergic individuals fear coming into any contact with food allergens. Reactions may occur when a food allergen touches the skin or is inhaled. For instance, skin reactions can occur when food allergens are present on the surface of a table or seat. Bakers who are exposed to high amounts of airborne wheat dust in their jobs can develop asthma, known as bakers asthma. Airborne allergens are released when peanuts are shelled, a package of powdered milk is opened, or fish is cooked. Reactions to these types of exposures are usually mild and severe reactions rare. Recognizing and avoiding situations that increase exposure to skin or airborne allergens will help to decrease risks and prevent or minimize a reaction.

Some allergic individuals become panicked if they just smell a food they are allergic to. But sitting near a food allergen and smelling it does not put an allergic individual at risk. When an allergic individual is near someone who is eating a peanut butter sandwich (or other allergenic food) or the smell of that food is very strong, there is little risk of allergenic proteins being released into the air because aromatic oils (not the protein) carry the smell. This type of situation is a low risk. But if allergenic food dust or protein is released into the air—which can happen when bags of peanuts are opened or shelled, foods are cooked, or dry forms of food (flours or dry milk powder) are being used in the baking and cooking process—allergy risks increase because allergenic proteins become airborne. If these proteins become airborne outside, a reaction will not usually occur because the open air disperses the allergen. But if they become airborne in closed spaces or where air is being recirculated, as may be encountered in a restaurant or on an airplane, the risk for a reaction increases. Although a reaction usually is mild if it does occur, a severe reaction is possible. When a severe reaction does occur, it is typically triggered by inhaling a large dose of the allergen all at once (which may occur when working in the kitchen of a fish restaurant) or exposure is prolonged (such as when traveling on an airplane and unable to leave the area).

In the case of skin contact with an allergenic protein, developing skin symptoms at the area where skin touched the food allergen is the typical reaction. Some allergic individuals may develop skin rashes when dining out after touching allergen residues accidentally left on a restaurant seat or table. One study of thirty children with a history of severe peanut allergy found only skin reactions occurred when peanut butter was rubbed on the skin. None of the children experienced a severe reaction (Sicherer, 2006). Most research validates this study, finding that allergen ingestion is the main method of transmission for severe reactions.

Food allergen exposures can also occur in very unexpected ways. Kissing is one such concern. If someone eats an allergenic food and then kisses a child on the check, redness of the skin may occur with no other symptoms. Passionate kissing, however, can transfer allergenic proteins that are then ingested and trigger a severe reaction. Using peanut butter, researchers measured the amount of peanut allergen in saliva over time. They found that, in most people, the allergen was gone by one hour. However, one person in the study was not allergen-free until four and one-half hours later. Brushing teeth or chewing gum did not always remove the allergen and could not be relied on to decrease this type of risk (Hallett, 2002). Therefore, adults, teens, and young adults are advised to always be open and educate their dates about their food allergy and the risks they encounter. Although difficult to do, it is absolutely essential to ask if an allergenic food was eaten prior to their date. If yes, then it is necessary to refrain from kissing for at least several hours. A worthwhile date will be understanding and put safety first. Take the case of a fifteen-year-old girl from Canada who had a peanut allergy. Her boyfriend had eaten peanut butter before visiting her. After kissing, this young girl suffered a severe reaction and subsequently died. Although the coroner later ruled there were other factors that contributed to her death, a severe reaction to the peanut allergen did not help to keep her alive (Laino, 2006, http://WebMD.com).

Participating in sporting events is another situation in which food allergens are usually not even thought about. While most teenagers do not expect to be exposed and usually do not carry emergency medications with them to sporting events, accidental exposures to allergenic residues can occur when cups, straws, or water bottles are shared. Sometimes allergenic snacks are on hand that may increase risk for a reaction. Coaches must be aware of food allergy risks and have emergency medications always available when a team member has a food allergy.

Food proteins are able to make their way into the bloodstream. This fact makes using donated blood risky. When blood is donated, red blood cells and the serum portion of blood are separated. Food proteins, in extremely small amounts, are sometimes found in the serum portion of blood. While only red blood cells are transfused, any food protein in the serum can contaminate them. There is only one known case where a peanut allergy was transferred to the recipient during a blood transfusion (Arnold, 2007). In this case an eighty-six-year-old woman with no previous history of food allergies received a blood transfusion in 2007. A nineteen-year-old woman who had a peanut allergy had donated this blood. Two days after receiving this transfusion, the older woman experienced an allergic reaction after eating a muffin that contained nuts. Skin tests a week later showed higher than normal levels of peanut specific IgE immunoglobulins. Three months after the transfusion, her IgE levels did return to normal, and she no longer experienced an allergic reaction when eating nuts. While a very rare possibility, the risk is still there.

Organ transplants have also been implicated in transferring food allergies. A sixty-year-old man, who received a liver organ transplant from a fifteen-year-old allergic to peanuts, developed allergies to cashews, peanuts, and sesame seeds (Phan, January 27, 2003). This study concluded that all organ donors should undergo allergy screening and advice about avoiding food allergens. Although the possibility of passing a food allergy to another exists, risks are still very low.

Using cosmetics, moisturizers, shampoos and conditioners, and skin care products, and toothpastes are more risky. Many of them contain food proteins as ingredients, and labeling laws in most countries do not require them to be disclosed by the manufacturer. Some manufacturers will voluntarily list ingredients, but more often than not consumers must call them directly to check if a product is "allergy safe." Using any of these products requires vigilance on the part of allergic individuals. Often contact dermatitis is the only reaction, but cases of anaphylactic shock have been known to occur, depending on the ingredient and the allergy.

Alcoholic beverages may present a risk as well. Besides the obvious possible allergies to grains used in making beers, some alcohols use clarifying agents (which makes the alcohol clear by removing any suspended materials) in their processing methods. Wines many use gluten or gelatin. Liquors may use egg or fish proteins in their clarifying process. Some liquors contain nut proteins. Label reading, when possible, is a must. But more often the manufacturer must be contacted to identify any potential food allergens in their products. Although a reaction to alcohol is rare, the possibility exists.

Other craft or household products may contain food allergens. Modeling dough often includes wheat, which can cause skin reactions in those with a wheat allergy. Risk is generally low and the reaction typically a mild dermatitis. However, the potential for many compounds and ingredients in our physical environment to trigger allergic reactions exists. Those who live with food allergies or hypersensitivities are always at risk and must always be vigilant and prepared at all times to deal with unexpected reactions.

6

Living a "Normal" Life

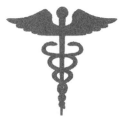

Living with a food allergy or hypersensitivity can turn an ordinary life upside down. The simple act of eating can become stressful or turn into a deadly experience. The psychological effect food allergies can have, along with tips and coping strategies for living with them in the "real world," are discussed in this chapter.

PSYCHOLOGICAL EFFECTS OF FOOD ALLERGIES

Individuals who experience adverse food reactions are frequently afraid to eat or to even come into contact with food allergens. Both children and adults become anxious about trying new foods. Some lose interest in eating altogether. Parents and caregivers may feel guilt because they feel responsible for "giving" their child the allergy. Family members often become frustrated or resentful because they must be extra cautious at home, cannot have their favorite foods in the house, rarely eat out, or decrease travel and social activities. Siblings at times may become upset with the extra attention an allergic child may receive. All family members and even the allergic individual themselves may experience anger, anxiety, depression, fear, frustration, sadness, and stress. All of these feelings are normal, but they can be overwhelming and, for some, crippling. So is it even possible for someone with adverse food reactions to live a "normal" life?

Realistically, food allergens cannot be completely avoided. Food allergens masquerade by unrecognizable names, show up in the most unexpected places, or are "hidden" in the environment. Despite all the best precautions taken to avoid them, adverse reactions do occur. Fear of these reactions can become debilitating and deprive an individual of an enjoyable and healthy life. Take the case of Melanie, a teenager who is allergic to peanuts. Her fear of having a reaction made her very anxious and stressed about eating new foods. Limiting herself to just a few "safe" foods, she unnecessarily lost weight. Her anxiety also affected her social life. One day while eating lunch with a friend, who happened to be eating potato chips, Melanie suddenly declared they smelled funny. Looking at the food label, she found the potato chips contained peanut oil. She immediately began to experience symptoms that included difficulty breathing, a racing heart, and profuse sweating. Treated for an allergic reaction, even though she never ate any of the chips, it was later learned that the peanut oil was highly processed and did not contain any peanut protein that would have triggered a "true" reaction. Melanie's anxiety and fear of a reaction actually triggered a panic attack, which has symptoms very similar to those of an adverse food reaction (Sicherer, 2006).

Psychologists report symptoms of depression and stress frequently begin to affect children between the ages of seven and ten, as they begin to realize the serious consequences that food allergy reactions can bring about. Fear of adverse food reactions may engender anorexia nervosa, avoiding social occasions, depression, headaches, insomnia, limited intake of foods, nutrient deficiencies, obsessive hand washing, panic attacks, stress-induced vomiting, and weight loss. Parents and caregivers are just as prone to stress and anxiety as well. Asthma, colds, or hay fever symptoms may cause them to become overly protective, overreact, or panic. When dealing with food allergies, the first instinct is to ban a food completely from the home. But these "precautions" do not teach the important lesson that it *is* possible to be around food allergens and *not* have a reaction.

Psychologists advise that daily life must be kept as normal as possible for those living with food allergies. Dining out, sleepovers and play dates, socializing, and traveling should all be included, not avoided. Some individuals report that talking over their fears with loved ones or parents, and then moving on and not dwelling on them, helps them to put their food allergies into proper perspective. Children and adults can also take control by being proactive through educating others, making their own foods or snacks, reading labels, and *always* being prepared with emergency epinephrine and medications for unexpected exposures. The realistic goal is to control the food allergy, not let it control them.

When children experience fear toward trying new foods, behavioral programs are one effective way to overcome this fear. Parents can use sticker charts with age-appropriate rewards when the child tries a new food. But this simple behavioral plan may not work for all children and certainly not for adults. At times it may become necessary for the individual or caregivers to use the behavioral services of a qualified physician, psychologist, or counselor to overcome and manage anxiety, eating disorders, fears, and frustrations. While some individuals require help with their fears, there are some general strategies all allergic individuals can follow that will help to minimize the risk of reactions.

COPING SKILLS AT HOME

Keeping allergenic foods in the house is worrisome. The amount of a food allergen required to trigger a reaction varies from person to person. In general, only one teaspoon of an allergenic food or protein may trigger a reaction. But high-risk or very sensitive individuals can experience a reaction when exposed to only one or two drops of milk or egg, one-half a peanut kernel, or breathing in only a small amount of airborne wheat flour or fish proteins. Some families completely ban the problematic food from the home. But learning how to reduce irrational fears and manage ever-present food allergens proves to be the best strategy for living as normal a life as possible. To learn these skills and stay safe at home it is important to:

- Read food labels and know the food lingo associated with a food allergen or additive.
- Label foods as "safe" and "unsafe" and store them in separate locations from each other.
- Designate allergen-free and safe eating areas in the home.
- Always wash hands before and after eating.
- Scrub down counters, tables, and utensils to minimize cross-contamination.
- Practice proper food preparation techniques and airborne allergen precautions.

Read Food Labels, Label Foods as "Safe" and "Unsafe" and Store in Separate Locations

Becoming familiar with the different names food allergens can go by and checking ingredients on food labels are extremely important when trying to minimize accidental exposures. Safe and unsafe foods should be labeled as an extra precaution and kept in separate areas in the kitchen pantry or refrigerator. Computer-generated labels that are customizable, ready-made food allergy labels (resources where they may be purchased are listed on the Food Allergy & Anaphylaxis Network [FAAN] website), or colored stickers may be used to label foods. Labels are especially helpful for children because it allows independence while keeping them safe as much as possible.

Designate Allergen-Free Areas

Allergen-free areas in the home, such as "allergy-free" dining table seating assignments and designating a room where no foods are allowed, can provide a safe place to go and ease of mind to someone with food allergies. These "allergy-free zones" reduce the chance that unsafe foods will be shared or that crumbs and spills will trigger an unexpected reaction. It is important to educate all family members about specific food allergy rules in the home and strictly enforce them.

Wash Hands Before and After Eating

Washing hands is an important habit before and after eating for everyone. It can prevent accidental contamination by removing potential allergens that may cause a reaction as well as help to prevent illnesses. A 2004 study by John Hopkins (Perry, 2004) discovered that most household dish soaps and cleaners remove enough peanut allergen to prevent adverse food reactions. Smearing peanut butter on the hands of subjects in the study, researchers used dishwashing liquid, Formula 409® cleaner, antibacterial hand sanitizer, Target brand cleaner with bleach, and plain water to wash their hands. The dishwashing liquid, Target brand cleaner, and plain water all adequately removed tiny traces of Ara h 1 (a major protein allergen in peanuts that causes severe reactions). But antibacterial hand sanitizer actually left residual allergens behind, showing hand sanitizers are risky and should not replace hand washing for individuals with food allergies.

Scrub Down Counters, Tables, and Utensils to Minimize Cross-Contamination

Cross-contamination is a concern when allergenic foods are kept in the home. Food preparation areas, cutting boards, knives, spoons, measuring cups, mixing bowls, spatulas, and other cooking utensils must always be properly cleaned so that no trace of food allergens remain. Cleaning tips in the home include:

- Thoroughly clean all counters, tables, and food preparation areas with hot water and soap or commercial detergents.

- Use two different sponges to mop up spills and wash dishes. One sponge should be designated allergen-free and kept in a separate location where accidental contamination cannot occur.
- Prerinse dishes and utensils before washing in hot, soapy water or in a dishwasher. When removing clean dishware and cutlery from the dishwasher, it is important to thoroughly inspect them for cleanliness, especially wire whisks, beater utensils, and other hard to clean dishware because they can easily trap food scraps.
- Carefully and thoroughly clean all pots and pans. Prerinse and scrub them before placing into the dishwasher.
- Frequently wash dishtowels, rags, etc. in hot water and laundry detergent.
- Use vinyl or plastic tablecloths because they do not absorb spills and can be cleaned easily to remove food allergens. Tablecloths should always be washed with hot water and soap after every meal.
- Use extra care when grilling. Grilled foods are a particular risk because cross-contamination can occur easily if a safe food (i.e., plain chicken) is grilled next to an unsafe food (i.e., chicken marinated in a peanut sauce) by spatters that occur when high heat is used. Allergen-free foods should always be grilled separately from unsafe foods. Wire brush scrubbing of a hot grill removes most unsafe allergen residue but is not 100 percent effective. One safe way to grill is to place a double-thick layer of aluminum foil on the area where the safe food is to be cooked. However, using a separate grill is the safest method for grilling allergen-free foods.
- Use clean serving utensils for every food served and never use only one utensil to serve all foods at the table.

Practice Proper Food Preparation Techniques, Including Airborne Allergens

Improper storage, preparation, cooking, and serving procedures can accidentally contaminate normally safe foods. To minimize this threat, all foods should always be stored in sealed containers. Safe foods should be stored on their own shelf in the refrigerator and above unsafe foods so that spills or leaks do not contaminate them. When airborne protein allergens are released into the air, which happens when foods are steamed or cooked at high heat on an open stove or baked goods are being mixed, it is important to:

- Cook the allergen-free meal first. Cover and remove this meal from the area before cooking any foods that have food allergens.

- Never reuse cooking oils. When foods are cooked in oils, protein is released from the food and left behind. Subsequent foods cooked in the same oil can then become cross-contaminated.
- Use clean utensils for each separate ingredient added or mixed into a recipe.
- Keep the allergic individual at a safe distance from the food preparation or cooking area. A distance of at least five or six feet has been reported as safe.
- Turn on or install an exhaust fan over the stove.
- Allow at least thirty minutes for the air to clear before allowing the allergic individual to enter the kitchen or room again.

Everyone who lives with an allergic individual needs to be educated about the allergy, the typical symptoms and potential for severe reactions, where to find the food allergy action plan and emergency kit, and what to do during an actual emergency. Practicing how to give an epinephrine injection and posting emergency numbers in a central location can also save time during an emergency when every minute counts. Babysitters, family members, and neighbors should be educated about the food allergy and what to do during an emergency in case their help is needed.

MANAGING THE SUPERMARKET

Food-labeling laws in Australia, Canada, New Zealand, and western Europe are very strict and helpful for consumers with adverse food reactions. In many respects, they are much more stringent than in the United States, but food labeling laws in the United States are making progress. The Food Allergen Labeling and Consumer Protection Act of 2004 (FALCPA) was implemented in the United States in January 2006. Prior to this law, detecting food allergens in packaged and processed foods was very difficult for consumers. Food manufacturers are now required to list the eight major food allergens by their commonly recognized name that may be present in their food products and also provide a warning on the label if the item was made in a facility where cross-contamination is possible. A new law, implemented in August 2008, will also allow manufacturers to voluntarily label their product gluten-free if it contains less than twenty parts per million (ppm) of gluten. An example of allergy warnings on food labels in the United States and Australia are found in Figure 6.1. Although this is a step in the right direction for food allergy consumers, unidentified food allergens can still be found unexpectedly in supposedly "safe" foods.

Sample Allergy Warnings on Food Labels

In the **United States**

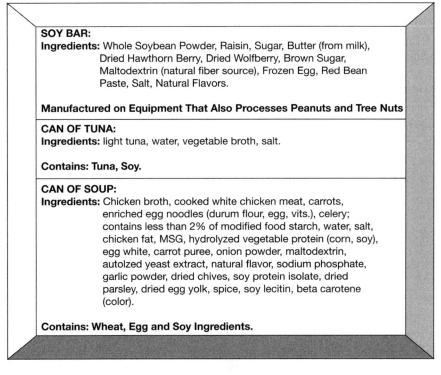

SOY BAR:
Ingredients: Whole Soybean Powder, Raisin, Sugar, Butter (from milk),
Dried Hawthorn Berry, Dried Wolfberry, Brown Sugar,
Maltodextrin (natural fiber source), Frozen Egg, Red Bean
Paste, Salt, Natural Flavors.

Manufactured on Equipment That Also Processes Peanuts and Tree Nuts

CAN OF TUNA:
Ingredients: light tuna, water, vegetable broth, salt.

Contains: Tuna, Soy.

CAN OF SOUP:
Ingredients: Chicken broth, cooked white chicken meat, carrots,
enriched egg noodles (durum flour, egg, vits.), celery;
contains less than 2% of modified food starch, water, salt,
chicken fat, MSG, hydrolyzed vegetable protein (corn, soy),
egg white, carrot puree, onion powder, maltodextrin,
autolzed yeast extract, natural flavor, sodium phosphate,
garlic powder, dried chives, soy protein isolate, dried
parsley, dried egg yolk, spice, soy lecitin, beta carotene
(color).

Contains: Wheat, Egg and Soy Ingredients.

In **Australia**

INGREDIENTS
Sugar, Full Cream Milk Powder, Wheat Flour, Cocoa Butter, Vegetable Fat
(Antioxidant [309]), Cocoa Mass, Cocoa, Emulsifiers (Soya Lecithin, 476),
Yeast, Raising Agent (Sodium Bicarbonate), Salt, Flavors, Glucose Syrup
(Derived From Wheat or Corn). Made on Equipment That Also Process
Products Containing Nuts. Contains 70% Chocolate and 30% wafer fingers.

Figure 6.1. Sample Allergy Warning on Food Labels [Jeff Dixon].

Food manufacturers in Europe list all ingredients in a product. However, food manufacturers still follow the 2 percent rule in the United States. This rule allows ingredients in small amounts (2 percent or less of total weight) to be exempted from the food label list of ingredients. The label may read "contains x% or less of a specific ingredient" at the end of the ingredient listing, but exceptions are allowed to this rule. Therefore, ingredients in insignificant amounts, such as "x parts per million," are not required to be listed and ingredients considered to be flavors or spices are not required to be specifically labeled as to what they are. These exceptions are allowed to protect the food manufacturers' proprietary rights to their "secret" ingredient(s). This rule can cause problems for those who are highly sensitive to a food allergen or additive.

In 2000 a study of food manufacturer inspections in Minnesota by the United States Food and Drug Administration (USFDA) revealed some disturbing findings. Approximately 25 percent of food manufacturers failed to label food products properly or accidentally cross-contaminated food products processed in their facilities. Almost 50 percent of companies also did not check their food labels to be sure ingredient listings were accurate (USFDA, 2001, Food Allergen Partnership). So what does this mean for those who suffer adverse food reactions? Obviously, checking food labels is still important even though there is a possibility they are not totally accurate. The good news is that most food manufacturers want to protect their customers, but using caution and common sense and being prepared for an emergency when eating processed foods is paramount. Whenever purchasing an item that has been consistently safe, *always* check the label for ingredient changes. Also check manufacturer, government, and food allergy Web sites for changes, recalls, or reported problems.

Fortunately, many food manufacturers are much more aware of the serious consequences of food allergies today than ever before. They are increasingly educating and training their staff about proper cleaning techniques to minimize cross-contamination and voluntarily listing all ingredients, even those in minute amounts, which are exempt from the 2 percent rule. Most food manufacturers provide a phone number for consumer questions. Increasing numbers of small, independent food manufacturers are selling allergen-free products from facilities where cross-contamination is prevented.

However, food manufacturers are still fallible. When in doubt, always call a manufacturer before eating a food or just avoid it altogether. General guidelines to use in the supermarket include the following:

- AVOID bulk food bins. Cross-contamination risk is high and ingredients are rarely listed.
- AVOID deli meats. Cross-contamination risk is high. The safest sandwich luncheon meats are those cooked and sliced at home.
- AVOID nut butters. Different nut butters are often produced on the same production lines, so cross-contamination risk with other nuts is high.

- AVOID baked goods, donuts, and muffins. Different types of baked goods are displayed near each other, making it easy for nuts or items made with eggs or milk to contaminate other foods. Serving utensils or tissue paper used to handle them may also contaminate foods.
- AVOID mixed foods. Foods that include multiple ingredients sometimes have unexpected ingredients. Risk is very high for unknown ingredients.
- AVOID candy bars, baking pieces, chocolate bars, and other candies. Plain candy is often processed in the same facility as those that contain milk, nuts, and other allergens or on the same production line. Although the line is cleaned between food products, there is still the possibility allergen residues may still be present, which cross-contaminate subsequently processed food products.
- AVOID mixing safe and unsafe foods in the shopping cart. Placing allergen-free foods into plastic bags before putting them into the shopping cart will prevent the possibility of cross contamination from allergenic food spills that could occur.

RESTAURANTS

Dining in a restaurant or eating away from home is always risky. The potential for cross-contamination or being served a food containing food allergens is very high. A landmark case in Australia highlights the dangers of eating out. In 1991 a young woman dined at a Thai restaurant in Australia. She informed the restaurant of her peanut allergy, but she still suffered an anaphylactic reaction (most likely from accidental cross-contamination) that left her with permanent brain damage. A lawsuit, seeking 10 million dollars in damages, was settled in 2000 (RG, 2007, http://www.geekzone.co.nz/Jama/2782). Fortunately, many restaurants are beginning to take food allergies more seriously and increasingly work with their patrons to ensure an allergen-free meal. The following tips can help decrease the risk of a reaction when eating away from home.

- Review the menu, research menu items on the restaurant's Web site, and check allergy Web sites for restaurant recommendations or ratings before dining out. Every restaurant prepares recipes differently, so never assume a dish that is safe at one restaurant will be safe in another. Fast food restaurants are the exception because they follow standardized recipes as a rule. But there can be regional variations, so *always* ask what is in a meal and how it is prepared before eating it.

- Call the restaurant ahead of time (and at nonbusy times) to ask how food allergies are accommodated and specific questions about cleaning methods used, ingredients, preparation techniques, etc.

- Choose nonpeak days to eat at a restaurant, avoiding Fridays, Saturdays, and Sundays (busy days). Special meal requests are more likely to be honored and the time available to prepare an accurate and specially made meal.

- Choose restaurants close to home where the manager or owner may be familiar and will take a special interest in ensuring special requests are followed.

- When at a restaurant, always speak with the wait staff and manager (also the chef when possible) and explain the allergy, food limitations, and possible life- threatening reactions. Ask about ingredients and preparation methods before ordering any meal (e.g., do they use clean cutting boards and utensils for different food items to avoid cross-contamination? Is the same oil used to fry different types of foods?). Give them a preprinted allergy card, listing all food restrictions as a guide (resource listings available from allergy organization Web sites).

- Order menu items that are simply prepared, avoiding breaded items, soufflés, soups, and stews. Chinese, Thai, and Indian foods are risky for anyone allergic to fish, nuts, peanuts, and shellfish because they are common ingredients in these dishes. Besides adding these ingredients, meals may also be prepared with equipment and utensils that can possibly cross-contaminate "safe" meals. These types of meals are safest when prepared at home.

- Beware of "secret ingredients" or "chef surprises" that may include unknown ingredients. Peanut butter may be added for extra flavor in marinades, sauces, and cocoa mix. Butter is frequently added to grilled steak to make it extra juicy. Asian meatless dishes, such as spicy fried dishes with lemon grass, are usually made with wheat flour shaped like beef, pork, and shrimp or soybeans shaped to look like chicken. Eggs are used in some dishes or as glazes for baked breads. Soy protein and flours are frequently used in baked goods, such as pizza dough for Mexican pizza. Pine nuts can sometimes be found in strawberry sauces, salad dressings, and spaghetti sauces.

- Ice cream parlors are risky because nuts may be mixed together with other toppings or drop into ice cream tubs.

- Muffins frequently have ground or chopped nuts added for texture and flavor, posing an obvious risk. Muffins are the safest when prepared at home.
- Fried foods are always risky because cross-contamination possibilities are high. Restaurants frequently reuse frying oil to fry more than one type of food. Restaurants also tend to use cold pressed, extruded, or expelled oils, which usually contain more allergenic proteins (because they are not heated) that may cause severe reactions. *Always* ask what type of oil is used and what foods are cooked in it when considering fried food.
- If the experience is positive, express appreciation, tip well, and recommend the restaurant to others.

When eating at another's home or at informal gatherings, bring along a "safe meal" whenever possible.

TRAVELING TIPS

Traveling can expose an allergic individual to cross-contamination risks or people who may not realize the importance of diet restrictions required by food allergies. But traveling does not have to be prohibited if appropriate safety precautions are taken. Precautions include:

- Informing travel companions about food allergies, possible reactions, and how to manage emergencies.
- Bringing updated prescriptions and all necessary medications. Keep epinephrine injectors and other medications accessible at all times, *not* packed away in luggage that may be inaccessible.
- Avoiding food served on an airplane unless *absolutely positive* the food is free of life-threatening allergens. Immediate emergency medical treatment in the event of a severe reaction may not be possible while in the air. Some airlines offer peanut-free flights. Check with the airline for these flights or other ways to decrease possible risks before traveling. The Food Allergy and Anaphylaxis Network (FAAN) provides tips about flying safely with food allergies.
- Carrying "safe" foods and beverages from home or purchased in the airport in case of delays and to decrease risks of an adverse reaction.
- Avoiding food from candy or vending machines. These machines are very high risk for cross-contamination because allergenic protein residues may remain from other candies and snacks.

- Using caution with cruises. Cruise lines are like airlines and being at sea is not optimal when suffering a serious reaction. However, many cruise lines appear to be responsive to travelers with food allergies and have emergency medical care available. Be sure to talk with the cruise line before taking a trip and reviewing accommodations and emergency care options.

Above all, *when in doubt about a food or meal, don't eat it!*

SCHOOLS

Young children tend to outgrow their food allergies by the time they start school. However, fish, peanut, shellfish, and tree nut allergies rarely disappear. For those school age children with food allergies, each age presents different challenges. Very young children need caregivers and teachers to be vigilant about their safety. Older children can begin to take responsibility for their own safety, but classmates and teachers need to be aware and supportive of their needs. Most schools and parents of classmates are very supportive of students with food allergies. Taking a proactive approach in accommodating them while balancing the needs of all students is the norm rather than the exception. Yet, this isn't always the case, as a January 2008 *Harper's Magazine* article highlights (Broussard, 2008). This article expressed the opinion that food allergies are currently viewed as "a childhood epidemic" and the pro-education efforts of many of the food allergy organizations and parent groups adds up to "cultural hysteria." Although the author has a point that food allergies are not as prevalent as most think and that excess societal anxiety about them can lead to psychosomatic reactions that do more harm than good, education and heightened awareness about the seriousness of food allergies and support by others is still critically important and not one to be downplayed.

Schools have sometimes been reluctant to take responsibility for fear of lawsuits. But the Centers for Disease Control and Prevention (CDC) found in 2006 that 98 percent of schools kept information on students with severe food or other allergies and 77 percent of school food service programs had a written plan for feeding children with food allergies. Unfortunately, some parents have had to resort to lawsuits to gain support for ensuring their children remain reaction-free while at school or after-school activities. In the United States, the Individual with Disabilities Education Act (IDEA), Section 504 education plan, and the Americans with Disabilities Act (ADA) protect students with food allergies in the United States. These laws protect students with food allergies from discrimination and ensure a safe school environment. Some schools have banned peanuts, peanut butter, and tree nuts because the risk for cross-contamination or exposures is high. While most parents support a ban, those with children who do not have allergies sometimes ignore it or become resentful. Some argue against allergen-free schools because they promote a "false" sense of safety in a world that can never be totally allergen-free.

But for those school age students with food allergies, the following guidelines can help reduce the risks of having an adverse food reaction at school. FAAN also provides a Back-to-School Tool Kit (available on their Web site) to help parents.

- Consider the school's record for allergy safety. Public schools are required by law to provide a safe environment, including safety from a fatal food reaction. But this does not mean private schools aren't as concerned or all public schools accommodating. Research the school and learn about their track record with students who have food allergies before enrolling a student.
- Review school food allergy policies and whether a school nurse or other trained staff member is on site. Ask if the school educates and trains teachers, coaches, cafeteria workers, aides, and all who work with students about handling food allergies and what to do during an allergic reaction. Question if substitute teachers are included in training and equipped to deal with food allergies.
- Learn where students eat snacks and meals. Keeping foods out of the classroom is the safest option but may not be realistic in small schools. Ask if "allergy-free" classrooms or cafeteria tables can be designated and check to see if this rule is enforced.
- Ask how often desks, chairs, and tables are cleaned, how they are cleaned, and by whom.
- Question if students are required to wash hands before and after meals.
- Discuss emergency procedures—who should the student go to for help during an allergic reaction, who will stay with the student during a reaction, where emergency medications and the food allergy action plan are kept, who is responsible for calling 911, and what alternate staff member will take over if the responsible staff member is unavailable.
- Learn if food service workers are experienced in preparing meals that are allergen-free and avoid cross-contamination. If preparation methods are questionable, bringing lunch and snacks from home is the safest practice.

- If the student rides the school bus, ask if bus drivers and substitute drivers are trained about food allergies and giving emergency care.

Parents can offer to educate teachers, staff, and other parents about food allergies, the food allergy action plan, accidental exposures and cross-contamination, and steps to be followed during a reaction. Parents may find sending a personal letter to classmates about their child's food allergy and precautions that can be taken helps to improve support and willingness to comply. Field trips and after-school activities (sports, band, after-school programs, etc.) can also be especially risky because the environment is less controlled. Learn who is responsible for the student's safety and how emergency medications will be accessed if needed.

Every student with a food allergy should have a food allergy sheet with their picture, list of allergies and triggers, and steps to follow to prevent allergy exposures. Administration, food service personnel, and teachers should keep these sheets for reference. Occasional class or school parties can also be risky. When planned in advance, the student should bring their own "safe" snack and understand that foods cannot be shared. For unplanned parties, parents can work with teachers to keep allergen-free snacks available for such occasions.

Even when the schools are supportive, reactions can still occur. Take the case of Nathan, a nine-year-old on a field trip with his class (Stark, 2008, http://ABCNews.com). The school, teachers, and trip chaperones knew Nathan was allergic to peanuts. During the field trip he was accidentally given a lunch that included a peanut butter and jelly sandwich, trail mix, and a peanut butter cookie. Although Nathan knew enough not to eat the sandwich or trail mix, he thought the cookie was a sugar cookie and ate it. He suffered a reaction, no emergency medication was given and Nathan died a few hours later.

An increase over the past few years in the number of "deadly" bullying cases, where some bullies actually use allergenic foods as weapons, is also being seen among schoolchildren across grades six to twelve. Take the case of an eighth grader in Kentucky who was severely allergic to peanuts. A classmate "spiked" his lunch box with peanut cookie crumbs. A thirteen-year-old classmate was subsequently arrested on felony wanton endangerment charges (Cox, 2008, http://ABCNews.com).

Teenagers and Young Adults

As children become older, they are able to begin to assume responsibility for protecting and advocating for themselves. They should be repeatedly taught to avoid food triggers by learning to read labels, recognize allergenic foods, take appropriate precautions, and care for themselves during a reaction. However, teenagers are notoriously rebellious and known risk takers. This age group has the highest death rates from food allergy anaphylactic reactions. Many teens view having a food allergy as making them "different" at a time when they most wish to be just one of the "group." Unfortunately, teens can be cruel and tease those with food allergies. Sometimes this teasing is harmless, but sometimes it is intentionally dangerous. When dealing with teasing, the teen must be reminded that their safety is paramount above all other concerns, and the best way to handle the situation is to ignore it. If the teasing becomes dangerous, adults must get involved, and the teen must realize that including adults in the resolution of this type of problem is necessary and possibly lifesaving.

Food restrictions and precautions are an absolute necessity and teens must be reminded that they have a serious medical problem that cannot be ignored. Parents must begin to transfer the responsibility of safety over to their teens and talk about sometimes difficult topics, such as safe kissing skills, and carrying an epinephrine autoinjector and medications at all times. If parents and teens clash over this area, having the family doctor or allergist discuss the seriousness of the teen's food allergy with them may be the answer. Teens may also benefit from the FAAN program *Be A PAL (Protect A Life)*. This program educates teachers and classmates about food allergies, what they can do to help prevent them, and how to react when there is an emergency. It is available on their Web site.

Camp, College, Day Care, and Other "Away from Home" Situations

One recent and disturbing study completed by the University of Michigan Health System found many college students with food allergies ignored their food restrictions. Many intentionally ate trigger foods and only 43 percent always carried epinephrine (UMHS, 2008, *ScienceDaily*). Other troubling studies performed by UMHS indicated that grade-school students are frequently in school systems that are not properly prepared for food allergy emergencies or have no food allergy policies in place.

So what is the best way to still live life or let go of a child? When attending a camp, college, daycare, or other organization:

- Speak to the director of the food service to learn food allergy policies and accommodations.
- Ask to look at a menu before arriving for possible problems.
- Visit the kitchen to inspect food preparation practices and risks for cross-contamination.
- Be vigilant about menu or food preparation changes, getting to know the food service director and kitchen workers so food allergy safety is kept uppermost in their minds.

- Bring along safe foods and snacks.
- Educate everyone involved so that safety is always kept in mind and mistakes are kept to a minimum. Roommates, friends, counselors, teachers, and all involved on a regular basis should learn food allergy symptoms, what to do when a reaction occurs, and how to prevent exposures. Having a "buddy" who is vigilant and takes an interest in keeping the allergic individual safe is an effective safety plan.
- Keep an ample supply of food allergy medications on hand. Be sure they are clearly labeled with name and in the original packaging with prescription information. Check expiration dates.
- Carry an emergency kit and food allergy action plan at all times and be sure these are also provided to appropriate staff members.
- Review basic symptoms, treatments, and prevention strategies. Stress the importance of telling others if a reaction is occurring immediately and *never* to drive oneself to the hospital or handle the reaction alone.
- Discuss common scenarios that could happen and how to handle them. For instance, talk about what to do if a reaction occurs when at the movies with friends and ways to prevent this.
- Wear medical alert jewelry or carry identification about the allergy at all times, even if it seems unnecessary.
- Above all else, use common sense, be extra cautious, and don't take unnecessary or foolish risks.

Bottom Line

Ultimately, children, teens, and young adults need to be proactive about their safety and realize that precautions and being prepared are a necessary fact of life. The Food Allergy Initiative (FAI) Web site, along with other food allergy organization Web sites, provides sound and helpful advice about living with food allergies and allergy research. An essay written by a teenager with food allergies, posted on the FAI Web site and reprinted in the sidebar, sums it up best. As this teen put it when discussing the discovery of her food allergies, her parents' help, and her journey to independence, "On July 4, 1989, at the age of two, I innocently stood on a stool watching my grandmother scramble eggs. Within a few minutes I was covered in hives. . . . Thus began a journey that we would experience together, but in the end would ultimately be mine alone." This is true for all who have food allergies or hypersensitivities, whether young or old.

Essay from a Food Allergic Teenager

July 4th is the day that we traditionally celebrate our freedom and independence. For my family and me, this was the day that we realized the severity of my food allergies. On July 4, 1989, at the age of 2, I innocently stood on a stool watching my grandmother scramble eggs. Within a few minutes, I was covered in hives from head to toe, my eyes closed shut, and I was gasping for air. Since we were visiting Long Beach Island, N.J., an ambulance had to come from the main land and rush my family and me to the nearest hospital. I was given a shot of adrenaline on route and my parents nervously waited at the hospital for many hours until I was stable and able to leave. Since I have no recollection of this event, I can only imagine how terrifying this was for my parents. Thus began a journey that we would experience together, but in the end would ultimately be mine alone.

It was not long after leaving Long Beach Island that I found myself in Dr. William Davis' office at Columbia Presbyterian Hospital in New York City. It was there that we learned the full extent of my food allergies, which includes eggs, tree nuts, peanuts, fish, and shellfish (lobster and shrimp being the most serious). At a young age, it was easy for my mother to monitor what I could and could not eat. She would be the one constantly checking the labels of food and packing me with safe snacks. I was known for my plastic baggies filled with teddy grahams and mallomars, and I was the only child in the entire school who brought their lunch each day. But instead of feeling isolated or different, my friends and teachers were supportive and curious to learn more about my food allergies. Every morning in primary school, when my gym teacher would take me out of the car, she would always ask me what I had for lunch that day. My lunch menu did not vary much; it consisted of turkey, Gatorade, Jell-O, and Vienna Finger cookies. My friends thought it was great that I had "cool" lunch boxes and could choose what I wanted to eat each day. At my closest friends' homes, safe snacks were kept for me to enjoy during a play date. My friends often loved telling their parents about my food allergies. They'd say "Oh Mom, make sure that you serve something that is safe for Brooke." If anything, my allergies were making me stand out in a good way. I know my parents worried about me (they still do), but I had to make safe food choices on my own. My parents made sure I lived by the mantra "when in doubt, do without." They insisted that I wear my MedicAlert bracelet, carry a safe snack, and have Benadryl and an EpiPen with me at all times.

Generally, I ran into very few food issues, but unfortunately there were some surprises that took place. One of the first incidents that occurred was when I was 7 or 8, and I ordered a hamburger that had been made with eggs. We did not think to ask what was in it, since eggs in a hamburger is rather unusual. But this taught that me that you have to ask questions no matter how plain the food is and no matter how many times you have previously eaten it. I was extremely nauseous after one bite, but I learned a valuable lesson that you can never be too careful. Unfortunately, there were other incidents that I stumbled upon. At a pizza restaurant, we specifically asked the waiter if there were eggs in the pizza dough, and he assured us that there were not. After one bite I was nauseous and vomiting, and luckily eggs are not the most serious of my food allergies.

Most kids love birthday cake, doughnuts, and brownies, but I was the one who was never able to try those foods. In 4th grade I wrote a story entitled What Does a Brownie Taste Like? I won an award for the story, and my mom till this day tells me that it broke her heart to read the essay. Since then my mom has made it her mission to create more home-made baked goods for me. Together we found an egg-free cookbook, which enhanced my love of baking and enabled me to try many new muffins, breads, and cakes. In recent years I sought the help of a nutritionist to provide an even greater variety of foods. Because of my expanding menu, I am able to vary my food choices when I travel and dine.

With age comes responsibility and I had to learn at an early age that it was imperative for me to be my own advocate. My "independence" began when I was 8 years old, when I attended an 8-week sleep away camp in the Berkshires for the first time. There I lived and ate without the help of my parents for 8 summers. The sleep-away camp was informed about my life-threatening food allergies and always had a plethora of food options for me. I had a chef who was sensitive to my needs and who always had separate food for me to eat. I was able to give the camp a list of the foods I enjoyed for breakfast, lunch, dinner, and snacks. I was the only camper who was able to walk up to the food counter and ask for whatever I wanted. (My allergies also enabled me to eat tasty food instead of the sometimes nasty food the other campers had to eat). When I was a younger camper, it was quite intimidating to walk up to the counter where all the other counselors were. I was often told that I had to sit back down because "no campers were allowed," but I knew that I had to be my own advocate and tell the other counselors that I had food allergies, and I had to have special food.

Following my summers at sleep-away camp, I traveled to Hawaii, London, and Paris during school vacations and went on a 4-week cross-country summer trip all without my parents. I was able to dine just like anyone else, though I did come prepared with bagged pasta in case of a food emergency. It was at this time that I designed a "safe-foods" allergy card. This hot pink card (the size of a normal business card), boldly listed all of my food allergies and stated that my allergies were life threatening. It was very empowering for me to create this card. If I even felt a waiter did not understand the severity of my food allergies, I knew I could not afford a mistake, so I would ask to speak to a manager or a chef. More often than not, I have found that waiters and chefs not only let me know what I can and cannot eat, but they often also take extra care when preparing my food.

At the age of 16, dining, traveling and dating have become regular activities without my parents. So when I entered high school, it was critical that all my friends understand the severity of my food allergies. My closest girl friends all know how to use my Epi-Pen if necessary and spot allergic reactions. In terms of dating, I have to somehow let the boy know about my allergies and tell him that eating at a Japanese, Chinese or seafood restaurant is not the ideal place for a date. To avoid an awkward first date I try my best to choose a restaurant where I have previously eaten. But probably the most uncomfortable topic I have to bring up on a date is that kissing cannot occur if he has eaten any kind of nut or fish. I bring this topic up nonchalantly, and the conversation usually turns out to be funny instead of embarrassing. So far it has not been an issue.

I must say that it was because my parents let me be independent that I never let my food allergies hold me back. My parents helped me find my voice, gave me the strength to be my own advocate, and to live by the mantra "when in doubt do without." I was encouraged at an early age to be an active participant and to experience life to the fullest. In addition to my academics, I play two varsity sports at school, am actively involved in student government, mock trial, key club, and community services. I have always considered myself a people person—outgoing, enthusiastic and friendly. And it has always been important to me to inform and educate people about the severity of food allergies. I have always enjoyed meeting with children and their parents to share my personal experiences about living with food allergies. I believe that children are at a disadvantage if their parents prevent them from doing normal "kid stuff" such as attending birthday parties, having play dates, and experiencing life away from home. My food allergies are only one part of me; they have never and will never control my life.

Brooke Jacobsen

Age 16

March 16, 2004

© Food Allergy Initiative, Inc. Reprinted with permission.

7

Is There Any Hope?

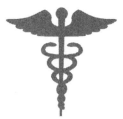

Progress is being made in the quest to learn more about what causes food allergies and how to treat them. Increased research efforts are directed at food allergies and hypersensitivities, with food allergy research studies growing from fewer than 100 in the 1970s to more than 1,000 in the twenty-first century. Beginning in August 2008 the United States, the National Institutes of Health (NIH), National Institute of Allergy and Infectious Diseases (NIAID), the Environmental Protection Agency (EPA), and various nonprofit food allergy organizations have committed research funds for a new food allergy research program. The "Exploratory Investigations in Food Allergy" program will focus on investigating the origin, epidemiology, and genetics of food allergy as well as encourage new investigators to enter this growing research area.

In Europe, concern over increasing food allergies and sensitivities throughout European countries led to the formation of the EuroPrevall Project in 2005. Scheduled to end in 2009, this multidisciplinary project is funded by the Global Allergy and Asthma European Network and includes seventeen European nations as well as Ghana, Iceland, and Switzerland. Since its inception, Australia, China, India, New Zealand, and Russia have joined as new partners. The goals of EuroPrevall are to improve the quality of life for people with food allergies, develop improved diagnostic methods that reduce the risk of food challenge testing, determine economic cost to individuals, families, and employers, analyze prevalence patterns of food allergy incidences in these countries, identify new and emerging food allergens, investigate the impact of environment, genetics, and the role of food processing, and develop a library of food allergens available to consumers and health care providers.

Many research studies are conducted, but how well a study is designed is critical for results to be valid and applicable. Studies about food sensitivities are particularly challenging because "allergy" symptoms can be caused by many other factors besides food and rely heavily on subjective information to make a diagnosis, and results are not always clearly linked to the study premise. Some areas investigated by food allergy studies in the past include:

- Characteristics of susceptible individuals.
- Determining specific foods that trigger reactions and symptoms.
- Frequency patterns of food allergies.
- Improved diagnostic and treatment methods.
- Natural progression of food allergies and patterns over time.
- Possible cures.
- Prevention strategies.
- The impact food allergies have on lives and society.

Medical research studies are divided into basic science studies, clinical studies, and translational studies. Basic science research studies are carried out in the laboratory using test tubes or animal experimentation. Basic food science studies typically test allergenic proteins. Although humans are not used, blood samples from individuals with or without food allergies may be used to test immune responses to allergens. Clinical research studies investigate individuals directly and include observational and epidemiological studies. Observational clinical studies monitor the experiences of individuals to a specific subject being studied. Food allergy *epidemiological clinical studies* focus on discerning what percent of the population is affected by food allergies, thus determining which are the most prevalent and the effectiveness of interventions. Translational research studies compare basic science studies to clinical studies for correlations. Discoveries in the lab are tested on humans, and the results are taken back to the lab for analysis. Results are then translated into promising new and innovative treatments or solutions when effective and practical.

All research studies must follow strict guidelines and protocols to ensure the relevance of the study while minimizing risk to study participants. Goals, objectives, and risks are explained to all participants (or parents if a minor child is involved). If test animals are used, humane treatment guidelines are followed. Review boards monitor studies to ensure all guidelines are followed and safety concerns enforced. Government agencies, such as the National Institute of Allergy and Infectious Disease of the NIH, often provide the majority of funds for research studies. But some funding also comes from the private sector, such as the American Academy of Allergy, Asthma and Immunology, the American College of Allergy, Asthma and Immunology, or the Food Allergy Initiative. Family-based organizations, such as The Food Allergy & Anaphylaxis Network, founded by parents and grandparents of family members with allergies, donate to food allergy research efforts as well. Thanks to these private donations, unusual and controversial theories (e.g., herbal remedies to treat food allergies, which are less likely to be supported with taxpayer money) can be investigated. The EuroPrevall Project is funded likewise via a consortium of government and private organizations.

Ongoing and new research work is also openly shared with colleagues around the world at yearly meetings. Once the results of a study are verified, they are reported to the public and other scientists. Media sources are often the first to report study results to the public, but the facts can be confusing or misleading. For example, study results in 2003 showed medicinal charcoal could bind peanut protein in the test tube. But media sources reported that activated charcoal could cure peanut allergies, drastically different from actual study results and potentially fatal for anyone trying this treatment.

CURRENT FOOD ALLERGY STUDIES

Food allergy studies completed in past years have at times provided contradictory results. Consequently, improved methods and study designs have been developed and implemented. Current studies focus on improving the accuracy of allergy testing while decreasing inherent risks. Yet, cause and effect is still a major drawback for all food allergy studies because so many other factors can produce similar symptoms. Some areas currently being investigated are:

- Using pure allergens, instead of food allergen extracts currently used, for skin prick and blood tests.
- Discovering new technologies to measure different IgE antibodies at the same time.
- Measuring mast cell activity to determine the degree of allergic responsiveness by improving cellular allergy tests.

New treatments are also in development. Some of these are:

- Developing safe immunotherapies (allergy shots) that will desensitize individuals to food allergens.
- Developing sublingual immunotherapies.
- Developing anti-IgE medicines, which currently show promise against peanut allergies.
- Evaluating the use of traditional Chinese medicine therapies.
- Using probiotics to stimulate the immune system.
- Developing DNA immunization techniques that stimulate the body to produce the allergenic protein it is allergic to, thereby rendering it no longer foreign and something to be combated.
- Developing epinephrine treatments for administration under the tongue.

Numerous study projects are already underway in 2008, with twelve investigators receiving grants in the United States that will tackle the problem of food allergies. The focus of these studies is to investigate which specific food protein components elicit allergic reactions, what influences trigger a severe response, unrecognized immune disorders that influence susceptibility for a food allergy, and the precise role between genes and the environment that may cause food allergies to develop.

POSSIBLE TREATMENTS OF THE FUTURE

Treatments that currently show promise are immunotherapies. Immunotherapy involves either activating or deactivating the immune system. Activating it makes the immune response stronger, while deactivating it makes it less likely to overreact and subsequently overrespond. Immunotherapy desensitization, also known as an allergy shot, is one form of immunotherapy that has been used successfully for environmental allergies, such as hay fever, for many years. Allergy sufferers are given shots of an allergen they are allergic to in increasing doses over a period of six to twelve months. Maintenance doses must then be given over a three- to five-year period for the desensitization to last. Approximately 80 percent of environmental allergy sufferers improve after receiving allergy shots.

Immunotherapy desensitization is a relatively new research area for food allergies because of the inherent risks for anaphylactic reactions. Results using food allergy shots have been varied, and those with a history of severe food reactions are unable to tolerate allergy shots. But there have been some reported successes along the way. One small, but well-designed, study in 1997 by Dr. Harold Nelson at the National Jewish Center for Immunology and Respiratory Diseases in Denver, Colorado (Nelson, 1997), established that peanut desensitization via allergy shots increased tolerance for peanuts in the diet. But a high rate of severe reactions, with one death resulting among the study subjects even though shots were carefully administered in an intensive care unit with emergency medical care available, also occurred. Although the study was stopped and is the only study of its kind to date, data results did show that peanut allergic reactions were less severe after desensitization. Although the risks of food allergy shots for peanut allergy are too high to make this a viable treatment option, new research into anti-IgE therapies may find that combining food allergy shots with an anti-IgE therapy may work as an effective and safe treatment in the future.

Another immunotherapy that is being investigated is the use of sublingual therapies. Sublingual therapies involve placing a drop of an allergen under the tongue, resulting in desensitization without significant risk for a serious reaction. Again, this method has had some success for pollen allergies with an "itchy" mouth as the most frequently reported side effect. Serious reactions have been rare. One study in 2005, using hazelnut extract sublingually, found almost 50 percent of study subjects with a hazelnut allergy experienced a increase in the amount of hazelnut allergen it took to trigger a reaction. Thus, tolerance to hazelnuts with little risk was significantly increased (Enrique, 2005). However, other studies have shown significant side effects or loss of tolerance for a food if this therapy was not maintained over time. Sublingual therapy is still investigational and still very dangerous at this time. But it continues to be studied, along with introducing allergens early in life as a preventive therapy.

Other immunotherapy treatments include DNA immunization techniques that use modified allergens for desensitization. This treatment involves modifying the protein structure of an allergen into a modified protein vaccine (similar to weak or dead bacteria or toxins used in vaccines that protect against infection, like tetanus). In altering the protein, the amino acid(s) responsible for triggering a reaction, such as the Ara h1, Ara h2, and Ara h3 peanut proteins responsible for adverse reactions, are removed. Once removed, repeated injections of the modified protein, recognized by the immune system but not capable of activating the allergy mast cells, teach the immune system to accept peanut proteins (or other allergenic food protein) again. Variations of this idea, such as breaking up the food protein into smaller pieces, altering food proteins via bioengineering, DNA immunization (in which the body begins to produce the protein it is allergic to and thus, no longer treats it as foreign), and allergy shots with food proteins from other foods in the same "food group" are also being investigated. So far these therapies look promising, but in animal studies only.

Anti-IgE antibody therapy involves the bioengineering of IgG antibodies (called a monoclonal antibody) that binds IgE, thus leaving IgE unable to bind to mast cells and basophils and preventing the release of chemical mediators, which in turn triggers a reaction. Clinical trials have been positive, and one treatment medication, omalizumab (known as Xolair®), has been approved since 2003 for the treatment of allergic asthma. Anti-IgE antibody therapy has also been shown to suppress inflammation and provide relief in individuals suffering with eosinophil-associated gastrointestinal disorders (EGID). One study, the TNX-901 study, investigated using IgG monoclonal antibodies (called TNX-901 in this study) to bind IgE in patients with peanut allergy. Study results found peanut tolerance was increased when high doses of TNX-901 were given. But the effect was short-lived and did not continue after treatment was over, with about 25 percent of study participants showing no benefit from the treatment (Leung, 2003). However, the results show promise for emergency treatment options after accidental ingestions and could be applicable for other food protein allergens. Other drawbacks of anti-IgE therapies include the fact that they are not a cure or vaccine, must be given by injection every two to four weeks, are expensive, cannot be given if circulating total IgE levels in the blood are high, and have not been studied or used long enough to assess long-term side effect risks.

Chinese herbal therapies originate back to the days of ancient China. Some of these herbal preparations, used for centuries, claim to treat food allergies. One study, using a concoction of nine Chinese herbs named Food Allergy Herbal Formula-2 (FAHF-2), found them to be effective in treating peanut allergy in mice (Kattan, 2008). But their mechanism of action is still not understood. Studies using these herbals are ongoing, and initial animal study results do look promising. But clinical trials with humans will eventually determine if they are truly effective or not.

Probiotic use is increasingly popular and appears to be somewhat effective in preventing food allergies and gastrointestinal disorders. Probiotics are live "good" bacteria normally found in the gastrointestinal tract. Their presence stimulates the immune system to respond protectively, providing positive health benefits. Improvements in atopic dermatitis symptoms have been seen when using probiotics. However, this has not been the case for food allergies yet. Overall, probiotics are safe for most people to use. But it must be remembered that this "good" bacteria is grown from milk, posing a risk for those with milk allergy. Individuals with a weak immune system or underlying diseases are at risk for developing a severe infection from the live bacteria. They may also cause unhealthy metabolic activity, excess stimulation of the immune system, or transfer of genetic information into cells.

Research is also looking into improved diagnostic methods such as allergen test kits for home use, blood cell and atopy patch tests, and improving current test methods for accuracy and safety. Clearly, much research still needs to be done, but testing and treatment breakthroughs look promising. With increased commitment to food allergy research, hope for those with food allergies and hypersensitivities has never been better.

FOOD ALLERGY RESEARCH RESOURCES

Checking government, research organization, and food allergy association Web sites for allergy research updates can be informative. Some of these organizations include:

United States National Library of Medicine and the National Institutes of Health

This government service provides information about current clinical trials worldwide via ClinicalTrials.gov. Their Web site is http://www.nlm.nih.gov/medlineplus/foodallergy.html#cat27.

The EuroPrevall Project

This is a multidisciplinary project funded by the Global Allergy and Asthma European Network. The first database of food allergens has been released and is posted on the Informall Web site. Information about the project and the database may be found at http://www.europrevall.org and http://www.informall.eu.com/WP5.htm.

American Academy of Allergy Asthma & Immunology (AAAAI)

An organization of medical professionals dedicated to the research and treatment of allergies in the United States, this group provides summaries of newly published peer-reviewed research in the *Journal of Allergy and Clinical Immunology*. Research summaries can be found on the website at http://www.aaaai.org/media/jaci.

Food Allergy Research and Resource Program

The University of Nebraska-Lincoln supplies *Allergen Online*, a peer-reviewed allergen protein database, and allergen study updates. A cutting edge resource that is extremely helpful, it is located at the Web site http://www.farrp.org.

The Food Allergy & Anaphylaxis Network (FAAN)

An organization representing parents, health care providers, government agencies, food and pharmaceutical companies, and schools worldwide, FAAN is dedicated to advocacy and education about food allergies. Committed to food allergy research, FAAN provides funds for research studies and updates on research efforts. Current study results can be found on their Web site at www.foodallergy.org/research.html.

The Food Allergy Initiative

This nonprofit organization raises funds for research efforts to cure and treat food allergies. Associated with the Mount Sinai School of Medicine in New York City, research efforts are based in the United States as well as internationally. Information on current research efforts may be found on their Web site at http://www.foodallergyinitiative.org/section_home.cfm?section_id=7.

The World Allergy Organization

This international organization includes seventy-seven regional and national allergy and clinical immunology groups. Dedicated to education, research, and training worldwide, research information can be found on their Web site at http://www.worldallergy.org.

These are some of the organizations dedicated to finding a cure for food allergies and hypersensitivities. More information about food allergy organizations may be found in Appendix D. For those who live with food allergies everyday, it is possible to live a "normal" life with food allergies and hypersensitivities. Caution, common sense, and vigilance must be a constant companion. But in the words of eighteenth-century English poet Alexander Pope, "Hope springs eternal in the human breast...."

Questions and Answers

Can someone with a milk allergy have an anaphylactic reaction if milk is spilled on him or her?

In general, contact reactions with small amounts of a food allergen are mild and only affect the area that the food allergen touched. For instance, if only a few drops of milk are splashed onto the skin of someone with a milk allergy, the typical reaction is mild and the reaction only at the site that came in contact with it. However, there are some exceptions to this. If a whole glass of milk is spilled onto that person, then a more severe reaction can occur. Likewise, if the milk allergen gets into the eyes, which is one of the most sensitive parts of the body and absorbs allergens the same as if it was eaten, then the allergen can get into the bloodstream and trigger a severe reaction. If the milk splashes onto the hands and the hands are not washed before eating another food or, the hand comes into contact with the mouth, then the reaction can turn severe.

Can an anaphylactic reaction occur if someone who just ate peanut butter kisses someone with a peanut allergy?

Studies find that food allergens are transferred through saliva from one person to another when they kiss passionately. Lip to lip or lip to cheek contact, although unlikely to cause a severe reaction, can also transfer allergenic proteins usually causing a mild skin reaction. Peanut protein residue can last up to four to five hours in the saliva, even if teeth are brushed. Therefore, it is best to avoid passionate kissing or sharing cups or straws for a few hours after eating an allergenic food.

Peanut oils can be listed as highly purified, cold-pressed, and some even peanut-free. Are any of these safe to eat with a peanut allergy?

Highly purified peanut oil is heat-processed and almost free of peanut proteins. Many peanut allergic individuals can eat these without experiencing a reaction. Cold-pressed peanut oil is not heated when processed, making the peanut allergens even more dangerous than usual because there are higher amounts of them present in the oil. Any advertising that states a peanut oil is peanut-free is probably not true and should not be trusted. Because it is difficult to know what type of peanut oil is actually used in many processed foods, it is best to avoid all forms of peanut oils. In restaurants, if vegetable oil is used, ask which specific one is used because peanut oil is considered a vegetable oil.

Is Yoplait® yogurt safe to eat if someone is fructose-intolerant? The ingredients don't list any fructose.

Even though fructose may not be listed on an ingredient label, it does not mean it is not present. Only the most common food allergens are listed on food labels. Beware of general terms, such as natural flavoring or starch. It is often necessary to call manufacturers to find out what the natural flavoring that is added is specifically. For example, in Yoplait® vanilla yogurt, the natural flavoring added is fructose, which must be avoided in the diet when fructose intolerant.

Should foods only be purchased from allergen-free manufacturers when living with a food allergy?

This depends on the food allergy or hypersensitivity and how sensitive an individual is to it. Most individuals can shop in a regular supermarket as long as they are careful to read food labels and understand terms and ingredient names for food allergens or additives. In general, it is safest to buy foods that are not processed and to cook or bake food items from scratch. For food allergens or additives commonly found in many convenience foods, or if an individual is extremely sensitive to a food allergen or additive, then using allergen-free manufacturers eliminates risk.

Should schoolchildren with allergies be put at allergen-free tables or should the school be declared allergen-free?

It depends on the age of the child and may not necessarily be the best policy for children in the long run. Very young children should be kept as safe as possible, so banning an allergenic food from the school may be appropriate.

But teachers and caregivers must still be vigilant and monitor all foods brought into the schoolroom. As children get older, it is important for them to take responsibility for their safety. No school or table can be 100 percent allergen free; accidental contaminations can occur, and an "allergen-free" school can give a false sense of security that is not possible in the real world. It is best to teach children how to remain safe and handle unexpected reactions while still fitting in with everyone else.

Is it true that having some of the food you are allergic to can help increase tolerance?

It is possible to eat foods that trigger adverse food reactions later in life. Children with egg, milk, soy, and wheat food allergies have a tendency to out-grow them by the time they are five (although this may occur at an older age than previously thought). This is why children are given a "food challenge" as they get older, which tests them with the food allergen to see if they are still allergic to it. However, it has been seen that a child who is no longer allergic to a food and then eats it only rarely, can relapse and become allergic to it again. Current research studies are also finding that those who are lactose-intolerant are able to tolerate milk when exposed to it in small amounts or when it is heated or cooked before consuming. Tolerance appears to increase over time if the food is kept in the diet and not avoided. However, this is not the case for a food allergy.

Do allergy shots, like those given for hay fever, work for food allergy?

"Allergy shots," also called immunotherapy, have been very effective against environmental allergens, such as those that cause hay fever. However, this has not been the case for food allergens. While one study shows some suc-cess in being able to decrease sensitivity to peanut allergens, a high percentage of study participants experienced allergic reactions. Thus, the effectiveness of allergy shots for use with food allergies has not been positive so far. Current research efforts are beginning to show that possibly combining anti-IgE thera-pies with allergy shots may lead to effective food allergy shots in the future.

Is it possible to eat chocolate if allergic to milk or eggs?

The only chocolate that is pure chocolate, nothing added, is baking choco-late and cocoa powder. All other forms have milk or eggs added into the mix-ture. They may also have nuts or be cross-contaminated by them. Some people can have an allergy to chocolate, but this is very rare and usually due to some other ingredient.

Is using hand sanitizer sufficient to clean hands from food allergens?

A study done at John Hopkins in 2004 discovered that most household dish soaps, cleaners, and even just plain water remove enough of peanut allergen to prevent adverse food reactions. But antibacterial hand sanitizer actually left residual allergens behind, showing hand sanitizers are risky and should not replace hand washing for individuals with food allergies.

I have a mold allergy and was told moldy or mold-ripened cheese makes it worse. Is this true?

According to the Food Allergy Research and Resource Program, there is no evidence that links mold-ripened cheese with mold allergies. Inhaling mold spores usually causes mold allergies. Although there may be a small amount of mold spores left on these cheeses, the digestive process would destroy it and they should not cause a problem.

I am lactose-intolerant and was told to avoid nondairy and dairy-free creamers. Why?

These ingredient terms do not mean foods are milk-free. Dairy-free is a term used by food manufacturers, but it has no FDA regulation in place governing its use. This food will usually have caseinates or whey, which indicates milk protein is present. Thus, it is unsafe for anyone with a milk allergy. Nondairy is a regulated ingredient term, but the regulation allows milk protein (casein) in the product. It too is not safe for anyone with a milk allergy. Some lactose-intolerant individuals can use a small amount of these products and not experience symptoms, but it depends on the individual.

I've been told that soy lecithin is safe to eat for anyone with a soy allergy. Is this true?

Most of the protein in soy is removed when soy lecithin is manufactured. Most individuals with soy allergies can eat it without experiencing adverse reactions. But not all the protein has been removed, and some people who are extremely soy sensitive do report symptoms. Therefore, it should be eaten with caution or avoided all together.

Are cytotoxic tests reliable for diagnosing food allergies?

Some alternative practitioners and labs offer cytotoxic testing (also called Bryan's test, the Metabolic Intolerance Test, or sensitivity testing), which claims that food sensitivities and allergies cause everything from acne to cancer to obesity and can be identified through their blood tests. The American Academy of Allergy, Asthma and Immunology (AAAAI), the largest group of allergists in the United States, has concluded that cytotoxic testing is unsuccessful when diagnosing food or inhalant allergies.

Appendix A

Nonallergenic Food Sources for Vitamins Found in Allergenic* Foods

Food	Biotin	Folate	Niacin	Pantothenic acid	Riboflavin	Thiamin	Vt. A	Vt. B$_6$	Vt. B$_{12}$	Vt. D	Vt. E
Asparagus		✓			✓						
Avocado	✓	✓		✓				✓			✓
Banana		✓						✓			
Beet greens							✓				✓
Broccoli		✓		✓	✓		✓				✓
Cabbage, Chinese							✓				
Canola oil											✓
Cantaloupe		✓				✓	✓				
Carrots,			✓				✓				✓
juice							✓				
Cauliflower	✓							✓			
Chic peas							✓				
Kale							✓				✓
Kiwi						✓					
Lentils			✓	✓				✓			
Lettuce, romaine		✓									
Lima beans			✓				✓	✓			
Liver, beef, chicken	✓	✓	✓				✓		✓	✓	
Mango			✓				✓				✓
Meat, lean			✓		✓			✓	✓		
Mixed vegetables							✓				
Mushrooms			✓	✓							

142

Olive oil

Orange,
 Orange juice

Papaya

Peach

Peas:
 Blackeye

Green

Split

Pepper, red sweet

Pork

Potato, baked in
 skin

Poultry

Pumpkin

Raspberries

Safflower oil

Salmon

Spinach

Squash, winter

Sunflower oil

Sweet potato

Tomato juice,
 paste,
 puree,
 sauce

Turnip greens

*Corn, egg, fish, milk, peanuts, rice, sesame, shellfish, soy, tree nuts, wheat.

Source: Linus Pauling Institute and Office of Dietary Supplements, NIH (online, September 2008).

Appendix B

Nonallergenic Food Sources for Minerals Found in Allergenic* Foods

Food	Calcium	Chromium	Copper	Iron	Magnesium	Manganese	Phosphorus	Selenium	Zinc
Apple		√							
Artichoke hearts					√				
Asparagus									
Avocado									
Baked beans									√
Banana		√							
Beet greens	√				√				
Black beans					√				
Broccoli		√							
Cabbage, Chinese	√								
Canola oil									
Cantaloupe									
Carrots, juice									
Cauliflower									
Chick peas				√					√
Cocoa			√						
Collards	√								
Duck			√	√					
Fruit, dried									
Garlic								√	
Grape juice		√							
Green beans		√							
Kale	√								
Kidney beans				√					√

146

Food								
Kiwi								
Lamb			✓			✓		
Lentils								
Lettuce, romaine								
Lima beans		✓		✓	✓	✓		
Liver, beef,		✓			✓	✓		
chicken		✓			✓	✓		
Mango						✓		
Meat, lean red	✓	✓	✓			✓		✓
Mixed vegetables						✓		
Molasses, blackstrap						✓		✓
Mushrooms								
Navy beans				✓	✓	✓		
Okra				✓				✓
Olive oil								
Orange								
Orange juice							✓	
Papaya								
Peach								
Peas:								
Blackeye,								
Green,	✓							
Split								
Peppers,							✓	
Black								
Red								
Sweet								
Pineapple				✓				

(continued)

147

Food	Calcium	Chromium	Copper	Iron	Magnesium	Manganese	Phosphorus	Selenium	Zinc
Pinto beans						√			
Pork				√					√
Potato, baked in skin		√	√						
Poultry		√		√			√	√	√
Prunes,			√	√					
juice			√	√					
Pumpkin				√	√				
Raspberries				√					
Refried beans									
Safflower oil									
Salmon									
Spinach	√			√	√	√			
Squash, winter									
Sunflower oil									
Sweet potato			√			√			
Tea, black,						√			
green						√			
Tomato juice,									
paste,				√					
puree,				√					
sauce									
Turnip greens	√								
Veg, dark leafy greens			√	√	√				
White beans	√			√	√				

*Corn, egg, fish, milk, peanuts, rice, sesame, shellfish, soy, tree nuts, wheat).
Source: Linus Pauling Institute (http://lpi.oregonstate.edu/infocenter) and Office of Dietary Supplements, NIH (http://ods.od.nih.gov/factsheets).

Appendix C

Nonallergenic Food Sources for Macronutrients, Fiber, Flavonoids Found in Allergenic* Foods

Food	Carbohydrates	Fiber	Flavonoids	Omega -3	Protein	Monounsaturated fatty acids
Apples		√ (w/skin)	√			
Artichoke		√				
Avocado						√
Banana		√				
Beans	√					
Berries, red, blue, purple			√			
Black beans		√				
Blackberries		√				
Broccoli		√	√			
Brussel sprouts		√				
Celery			√			
Chickpeas		√				
Chocolate			√			
Citrus fruits, juices			√			
Collards						
Dates		√				
Figs		√				
Fruits	√					
Flaxseed				√		
Grapes, red, blue, purple			√			
Guava		√				
Hot peppers						

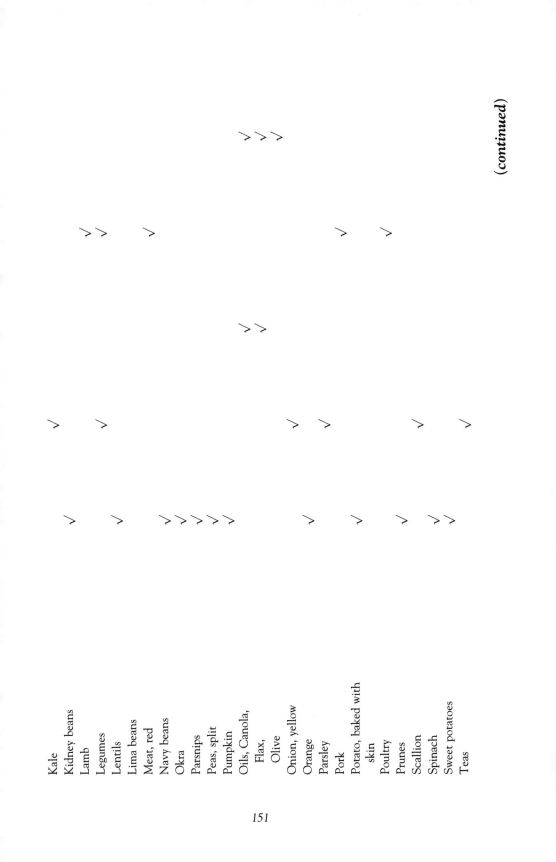

Kale
Kidney beans
Lamb
Legumes
Lentils
Lima beans
Meat, red
Navy beans
Okra
Parsnips
Peas, split
Pumpkin
Oils, Canola,
Flax,
Olive
Onion, yellow
Orange
Parsley
Pork
Potato, baked with
skin
Poultry
Prunes
Scallion
Spinach
Sweet potatoes
Teas

(continued)

Food	Carbohydrates	Fiber	Flavonoids	Omega-3	Protein	Monounsaturated fatty acids
Thyme			√			
Tomato paste		√				
Turnip greens		√				
Veal					√	
Vegetables	√					
Wine, red			√			
Winter squash		√				

*Corn, egg, fish, milk, peanuts, rice, sesame, shellfish, soy, tree nuts, wheat).

Source: Linus Pauling Institute (http://lpi.oregonstate.edu/infocenter) and Office of Dietary Supplements, NIH (http://ods.od.nih.gov/factsheets).

Appendix D: Resource List

The following resources provide accurate and valuable information about food allergies and hypersensitivities from reputable and reliable organizations.

AllAllergy.net: http://www.allallergy.net
Allergy & Asthma Network of Mothers of Asthmatics: http://www.aanma.org
AllergyKids.com: http://www.allergykids.com
Allergy UK: http://www.allergyuk.org
The American Academy of Allergy, Asthma, and Immunology: http://www.aaaai.org
American Academy of Pediatrics: http://www.aap.org
The American College of Allergy, Asthma, and Immunology: http://www.acaai.org
American Dietetic Association: http://www.eatright.org
American Gastroenterological Association: http://www.gastro.org
American Partnership for Eosinophilic Disorders: http://www.apfed.org
The Anaphylaxis Campaign: http://www.anaphylaxis.org.uk
Anaphylaxis Canada: http://www.anaphylaxis.org
Asthma and Allergy Foundation of America: http://www.aafa.org
The British Dietetic Association: http://www.bda.uk.com
Celiac Disease Foundation: http://www.iffgd.org

Celiac Sprue Association: http://www.csaceliacs.org

Center for Food Safety and Applied Nutrition: http://www.cfsan.fda.gov

Codex alimentarius: http://www.codexalimentarius.net/gsfaonline/index.html

Crohn's and Colitis Foundation of America: http://www.ccfa.org

Day Pharmaceutical Company: http://www.epipen.com

Dietitians Association of Australia: http://www.daa.asn.au

Dietitians of Canada: http://www.dietitians.ca

Food Allergy & Anaphylaxis Network (FAAN): http://www.foodallergy.org

The Food Allergy Initiative (FAI): http://www.foodallergyinitiative.org

The Food Allergy Kitchen: http://www.foodallergykitchen.com

Food Intolerance Awareness: http://www.foodintoleranceawareness.org

The Jaffe Food Allergy Institute at Mount Sinai: http://www.mssm.edu/jaffe_food_allergy

Gluten Intolerance Group of North America: http://www.gluten.net

HFI Laboratory at Boston University: http://www.bu.edu/aldolase/HFI

International Foundation for Functional Gastrointestinal Disorders: http://www.iffgd.org

Living Without Magazine: http://www.livingwithout.com

Medic Alert: http://www.medicalalert.org

New Zealand Dietetic Association: http://www.dietitians.org.nz

The University of Maryland Center for Celiac Research: http://www.celiaccenter.org

Verus Pharmaceutical Company: http://www.twinject.com

World Allergy Organization: http://www.worldallergy.org

World Health Organization: http://www.who.int/en

The following companies offer allergen-free foods.

Allergy Grocer: http://allergygrocer.com

Birkett Mills: http://www.thebirkettmills.com

Bob's Red Mill: http://www.bobsredmill.com

Cherrybrook Kitchen: http://www.cherrybrookkitchen.com

Divvies: http://www.divvies.com

Ener-G.com: http://www.ener-g.com

Food Matters: http://www.foodmatters-online.com

Gak's Snacks: http://www.gakssnacks.com

GlutenFree.com: http://www.glutenfree.com

Nu-World Amaranth: http://www.nuworldfoods.com

Gluten Free Mixes: http://www.glutenfreemixes.com

Grainworks: http://www.grainworks.com

Pangea: http://www.pangeaveg.com

The Sonnet Butter Company: http://www.soynutbutter.com
Tinkyada: http://www.tinkyada.com
Vermont Nut-Free Chocolates: http://www.vermontnutfree.com
Wellness Grocers: http://www.wellnessgrocer.com
Zing Bars: http://www.zingbars.com

The following websites provide information about nutrients and their food sources.

Linus Pauling Institute: http://lpi.oregonstate.edu/infocenter
Office of Dietary Supplements: http://ods.od.nih.gov/factsheets

Timeline

18th century	The method of variolation, used to protect the population from smallpox epidemics, was introduced into Europe from Istanbul.
1721	Lady Mary Wortley Montague introduced the method of variolation in England. Trial tests of variolation were first used on prisoners.
	Variolation tried in Boston, Massachusetts, by Rev. Cotton Mather and Dr. Zabdiel Boylston during a severe smallpox epidemic to prevent further deaths.
1722	The two daughters of the Princess of Wales in England were successfully protected from small pox using variolation. The practice became widespread throughout England after this, spreading into western Europe.
1757	Edward Jenner discovered inoculation. Inoculating an eight-year-old boy using pus from a cowpox boil, he later inoculated him with smallpox and successfully protected him against it. Jenner called this procedure vaccination.
1800	Vaccination became widespread throughout England and Europe, eventually replacing variolation.

1819	John Bostock was the first to describe the symptoms of allergic rhinitis.
1840	Variolation was prohibited in England because of its associated risks.
1869	Charles Blakely performed the first skin test to detect substances that trigger allergic reactions.
1877	Paul Ehrlich discovered mast cells and worked with Elie Metchnikoff on cellular immunity research.
1878	Louis Pasteur developed vaccines made from attenuated chicken cholera. These vaccines were successfully used to immunize sheep and cattle against anthrax.
1884	Elie Metchnikoff proposed the theory of phagocytosis in immunity. Also linked longer life with the use of acidophilus type bacteria, an early precursor of probiotics.
1885	Louis Pasteur developed the rabies vaccine and became a national hero in France.
1890–1892	Emil Adolph von Behring demonstrated circulating antitoxins against diptheria-conferred immunity. This finding represented the beginning of serum therapy, which treats an infectious disease with an injection of serum containing a specific antibody.
1897	Paul Ehrlich standardized diphtheria toxin and antitoxin serums.
1900	Paul Ehrlich discovered antibody synthesis, linking it with genetic responses to immunity.
1902	Charles Richet and Paul Portier invented the word anaphylaxis for the life-threatening symptoms triggered by allergic rhinitis (hay fever).
1903	Svante Arrhenius hypothesized antigen-antibody complexes are reversible and coined the term "immunochemistry." Nicolas Maurice Arthus was the first to describe local anaphylaxis, known as the Arthus reaction.
1906	Clemens Freiherr von Pirquet coined the term "allergy."
1908	Elie Metchnikoff and Paul Ehrlich awarded the Noble Prize for their research on cellular immunity.

1911–1914	Leonard Noon and John Freeman established the basis for immunotherapy, also called allergy shots.
1913	Charles Robert Richet awarded the Nobel Prize for his work researching the anaphylactic reaction.
1919	Jules Bordet awarded the Nobel Prize for studies on immunity, linking antigen-antibody-complement interactions.
1921	Carl Prausniztz-Giles, called the "Father" of clinical allergy, made many significant contributions in immunology research. He and Heinz Kustner discovered the passive transfer of hypersensitivity in 1921, eventually linking this with certain types of food allergy.
1930	Karl Landsteiner won the Nobel Prize for the discovery of human blood groups.
1935	Henry Hallett Dale awarded the Nobel Prize for the discovery of histamine and the development of the Schultz-Dale test for anaphylaxis.
1937	Daniel Bovet synthesized the first antihistamine drug.
1940s	Robin R.A. Coombs developed the Coombs' test, which detects immunoglobulin on the surface of red blood cells.
1942	Karl Lansteiner and Merrill Chase proved white blood cells are involved with contact and delayed sensitivity reactions, demonstrating passive immunity.
1948	Philip Hench and Edward Kendall discovered corticosteroids, effective in treatment for asthma, delayed, and immediate allergic reactions.
1950s	Astrid Elsa Fagraeus-Wallbom provided first observable evidence that immunoglobulins are made in plasma B cells.
1953	James F. Riley and Geoffrey B. West discovered the mast cell granule to be a major source of histamine in the body and its connection to allergy and inflammatory responses.
1963	Hypersensitivity classification system developed by P. H. G. Gell and Robin Coombs. The most widely used allergy classification system worldwide today, the *Gell and Coombs Classification System* defines six different classes of hypersensitive reactions.

1967	Kimishige and Terako Ishizaka discovered IgE antibodies and their connection as principal mediator in the allergic reaction. Their work is regarded as a major breakthrough in understanding the allergy response.
1972	Richard K. Gershon discovered the suppressor role of the T cell.
1975	Henry George Kunkel awarded the Lasker award for his work on immunoglobulins. Discovered the IgA antibody.
1977	Smallpox declared eradicated worldwide by the World Health Organization.
1980s	George Davis Snell awarded the Nobel Prize for discovering cell structures that regulate immunologic reactions.
	Baruj Benacerraf awarded the Nobel Prize for demonstrating that genes control the antigen response.
	Bengt I. Samuelsson awarded the Nobel Prize for identifying leukotrienes, which are mediators in allergy, asthma, and inflammation.
1990	E. Donnall Thomas and Joseph E. Murray awarded the Nobel Prize for their research on reducing the risk of organ rejection by the immune system.
2000	Cincinnati Children's Hospital Medical Center research team discovers eotaxin, a chemokine that controls food allergy reactions in the gastrointestinal tract.
2006	Researcher's at Cincinnati Children's Hospital Medical Center discovered the first gene associated with eosinophilic esophagitis.
2007	Claudio Nicoletti discovered food allergy susceptibility increases when the molecule Interleukin-12 (IL-12), produced by dendritic cells, is missing in mice.

Glossary

Allergen Any substance that triggers an allergic reaction. Food allergens are proteins that trigger the immune system to overreact, producing symptoms. Allergens may be airborne, contactants with skin or mucosa, or ingested. Some allergens are "hidden" from unsuspecting consumers when they are added to processed foods or through cross-contamination by contact with allergenic foods.

Allergic intoxication State of being poisoned by an allergen. Histamine and tyramine are two food substances that may cause allergic intoxications.

Allergy Hypersensitive response by the immune system to normally safe substances. **Food allergy** is an abnormal reaction by the immune system to food protein. Eight food allergens are responsible for approximately ninety percent of food allergy reactions worldwide. They include egg, fish, milk, peanuts, shellfish, soy, tree nuts, and wheat.

Amino acid Molecule that is considered a building block of protein.

Anaphylaxis Severe, immediate, and sometimes fatal systemic response to an allergen.

Angioedema Fluid leakage from blood vessels in the layers below the skin, which causes swelling and may produce abdominal cramping, breathing difficulty, welts on the face and around the eyes, and swollen lining of the eyes. Usually accompanies hives but can occur without them.

Antibody A protein manufactured by white blood cells that render threatening substances harmless.

Antigen Substance, usually a protein, that triggers an immune response resulting in antibody production.

Antihistamine Medication that counteracts the effect of histamine released by the body or via foods.

Arthus reaction Anaphylactic reaction that only affects one, not all, body systems.

Asthma Breathing disorder that causes coughing, difficulty with breathing, tightening in the chest, and wheezing. May be life-threatening.

Attenuated Weakened form of a living microorganism given as a vaccine to stimulate antibody formation and provide immunity.

Atopy Inherited allergy characterized by asthma, hay fever, or hives that develops when exposed to environmental antigens, usually through inhalation.

Atopic dermatitis Chronic skin disease characterized by itchy, inflamed, and red skin. Thought to be hereditary and often caused by foods.

Avoidance diets Eating plans specifically designed to avoid a food or substance that triggers an adverse reaction, while also balancing daily nutrients necessary for good health.

β-galactosidase Also called lactase, it is the enzyme that breaks down the milk sugar lactose in the gastrointestinal tract.

B-cells One type of lymphocyte that forms and matures in the bone marrow and is responsible for identifying invaders and defending against them.

Basophil A B cell lymphocyte that is activated during the immune response. Usually protects the body from bacteria and viruses but does respond to allergens.

Be A PAL (*Protect A Life*) Program Education awareness program developed and offered by the Food Allergy & Anaphylaxis Network. This program educates teachers and classmates about food allergies, what they can do to help prevent them, and how to respond during an emergency.

Bioengineered intoxications Plants, animals, or microorganisms that are altered genetically by inserting foreign genes into their genetic codes to increase desirable traits, disease resistance, and yield. Food allergies or other unintended outcomes may result. StarLink corn is one famous example of an altered corn plant that caused corn allergies in previously unaffected individuals.

Biphasic reaction Delayed response, after exposure to an allergen, anywhere from one to four hours after initial symptoms have subsided. In rare cases, symptoms can continue over a period of days.

Bradykinins Inflammatory mediator chemicals released during allergic reactions that trigger vasodilatation and contraction of smooth muscle.

Celiac disease See Gluten intolerance.

Cell-mediated reaction Reaction that occurs from an immune response by T cell lymphocytes. Also known as cellular immune response.

Chemical mediators Chemical substance in the body that acts on blood vessels and body cells contributing to the inflammatory response. Bradykinins, cytokines, histamine, leukotrienes, and prostaglandins are examples of chemical mediators.

Chemokine A cytokine produced in response to acute and chronic inflammation that activates white blood cells.

Crohn's disease Chronic and recurring inflammatory bowel disease characterized by inflammation of the small bowel. The colon may also be affected.

Cross-contamination Situation in which a normally safe food is contaminated by a food allergen from an unsafe source. This can occur during cooking, preparation, or processing.

Cytokines Inflammatory mediator chemical released during an immune response that triggers allergy symptoms.

Dendritic cells Immune cell with threadlike tentacles that ensnare antigens and present them to T cells for destruction.

Diverticulitis, Diverticulosis Digestive disorders. Diverticulosis is weakening of the colon walls, causing diverticula to protrude out and usually does not produce symptoms. Diverticulitis is inflammation and infection of the diverticula, requiring medical intervention.

Eczema Acute or chronic inflammation of the skin, characterized by extreme dryness and itching. May or may not be caused by a food allergy. Usually called atopic dermatitis when caused by a food allergy.

Elimination diets A strict meal plan that removes suspected allergenic foods and/or substances from the diet over a two- to four-week time period. Evaluation of symptoms is assessed after this time for improvement and typically followed by a food challenge to confirm diagnosis.

Emergency kit A kit that includes all prescribed medications and the *food allergy action plan* for treating severe allergy reactions.

Eosinophil-associated gastrointestinal disorders (EGID) Medical disorder characterized by inflammation and excess production of eosinophils in the gastrointestinal tract.

Eosinophil A type of white blood cell, also known as a leukocyte. Actively involved in the immune response.

Epinephrine A hormone that relaxes bronchioles in the lungs and acts as a vasoconstrictor and cardiac stimulant. It is administered by injection during severe allergic reactions to ease symptoms. Brands used for severe food allergy reactions are *EpiPen® Jr.*, *EpiPen®*, *Twinjet®*, and **Ana Guard**. *EpiPen® Trainer – Auto-Injector Training Device* is used as a practice tool for giving injections.

European Academy of Allergology and Clinical Immunology (EAACI) Nonprofit association of forty European organizations whose mission is to assess, collect, and disseminate scientific information. Proposed redefining an allergy as "a hypersensitivity reaction initiated by immunologic mechanisms" in 2001.

EuroPrevall Multidisciplinary project of seventeen European Union member states, plus Ghana, Iceland, and Switzerland, studying patterns, prevalence, and social impact of food allergies. Goals are to disseminate information and improve quality of life for individuals with food allergies.

Food action allergy plan A written summary of medical treatment steps to follow during a severe reaction.

Food additives "… all substances …, the intended use of which results or may reasonably be expected to result, directly or indirectly, either in their becoming a component or otherwise affecting the characteristics of food". Added to foods to decrease the risk of food spoilage, preserve and enhance flavor, or improve the physical appearance of a food. Some cause hypersensitivity reactions in sensitive individuals. Troublesome food additives include: Aspartame, Benzoates, BHA (butylated hydroxyanisole), BHT (butylated hydroxtoluene), MSG (monosodium glutamate), Nitrates and Nitrites, Parabens, Sorbate and Sorbic acid, Sulfites, and Tartrazine (FD&C yellow dye #5).

Food challenge Controlled allergy test under strict medical supervision that involves consuming a suspected allergenic food to confirm it as a trigger for allergic reactions. Performed using *double-blind, placebo-controlled food challenge* (*DBPCFC*) method or *Open challenge* method. Both methods can positively confirm a trigger food.

Food-dependent exercise-induced anaphylaxis (EIA) A rare allergic response, symptoms typically occur one to four hours after eating a trigger food *and* after any kind of physical exertion. The reaction *does not* occur unless both the trigger food and exercise are combined. There are three types of EIA: specific food EIA, non-specific food EIA, and medication or drug-dependent EIA.

Food intolerances Also known as metabolic disorders, anaphylactoid reactions, and idiosyncratic reactions, food intolerances are an inborn defect in food digestion and metabolism. The most common food intolerances include **lactose, fructose,** and **gluten** intolerances.

Food poisoning Illness caused by eating foods or drinks that are contaminated with bacteria, metals, parasites, prions, toxins, or viruses. Although it is *not* a food hypersensitivity or allergy, mild symptoms can be confused with them. Symptoms almost always affect the gastrointestinal system and usually occur from two to six hours after eating or drinking the infected food or liquid.

Food protein-induced entercolitis or proctocolitis (allergic proctocolitis) syndrome Medical disorder seen in infants, usually before three months of age, and children. Symptoms are bright red blood in the stool and prolonged projectile vomiting beginning one to three hours after drinking cow's milk or a soy protein-based formula.

Fructose intolerance, malabsorption Inborn defects in digestion and metabolism of fructose, a simple sugar. There are two distinct forms of defective fructose metabolism, Hereditary Fructose Intolerance and Fructose Malabsorption.

Gell and Coombs Classification System Hypersensitivity classification system developed by P. H. G. Gell and Robin Coombs in 1963. The most widely used allergy classification system worldwide, it defines six different classes of hypersensitive reactions. Type I hypersensitivity and Type IV hypersensitivity classes define adverse food reactions.

Gliadin Glycoprotein that makes up the protein gluten, which triggers hypersensitivity or allergy responses.

Gluten Protein in wheat that can trigger an allergic reaction in susceptible individuals.

Gluten intolerance Also called gluten-sensitive enteropathy or celiac disease, this inherited disease affects the small intestine and is frequently confused with wheat allergy. Although the immune system is involved, it is considered an autoimmune disease and not a food allergy because chemical mediators are not released in response to the gluten molecule.

Gluten-sensitive enteropathy (gluten intolerance, celiac disease) Inherited disease, frequently confused with wheat allergy, which affects the small intestine. Although the immune system is involved, it is considered an autoimmune disease and not a food allergy. Eating gluten causes the immune system to attack this protein and damage the inner lining of the intestine. Damage is reversible when gluten is strictly eliminated from the diet.

Gustatory flushing syndrome A harmless medical condition in which spicy or tart foods stimulate the auriculotemporal nerves, which control salivary and sweat glands along with blood vessels, in the face. Usual symptoms include facial flushing/ blushing or red spots on the cheeks that disappear quickly.

Heiner syndrome Rare disorder related to the pulmonary disease hemosiderosis. Occurs most often in children between the ages of six months to two years and a hypersensitivity reaction to the proteins in cow's milk.

Histamine Chemical present in B cells that is released during an allergic reaction. Triggers allergy symptoms.

Hives Also called urticaria. Extremely itchy, raised white areas surrounded by a reddened area on the skin. When a food allergen triggers histamine release, permitting fluid to leak out of blood vessels underneath the skin, hives occur. Hives can also be caused by anxiety, chemical reactions, extreme temperatures, irritations (like clothes rubbing directly on the skin), or viruses.

Hygiene hypothesis This theory suggests that living in developed nations, where cleanliness is an obsession and parasitic diseases are rare, ultimately creates an increased susceptibility to allergens. It is thought that excessive cleanliness forces an idle immune system to look for something to do by fighting harmless food and airborne allergens instead.

Hypersensitivity Abnormal sensitivity to a substance or food. These reactions are distinguished by whether IgE antibodies are produced or not. If IgE antibodies are produced, the reaction is classified as a food allergy or IgE-mediated food allergy. All other adverse food reactions, including food intolerances, food-related medical disorders, or food hypersensitivity are classified as nonallergic food hypersensitivities. There are immediate hypersensitivity reactions and delayed hypersensitivity reactions. In immediate reactions, symptoms occur within minutes. Delayed reactions can occur three to four hours after a reaction appears resolved.

IgE-mediated reaction Allergic response when an IgE antibody attaches itself to a threatening amino acid. Alerting the appropriate B cell to respond, the B cell then sprays the threatening amino acid with a chemical mediator, usually histamine, which triggers symptoms.

Immunoglobulin antibodies Group of closely related proteins activated during the immune response to threatening microorganisms and allergens. IgA, IgD, IgE, IgG, and IgM are antibodies in humans that fight specific types of microorganisms.

Immunology Science that studies the human immune system. Edward Jenner (1749–1822) conducted the first immunology experiment and is credited as both the founder of immunology and with introducing vaccination to the world.

Inflammatory mediators Special chemicals (bradykinins, cytokines, histamine, leukotrienes, prostaglandins) that fight inflammation and destroy potentially harmful allergens.

Inoculate Injection of a microorganism or toxin into the body to stimulate antibody production by the immune system, which in turn protects against future exposures to it.

Irritable bowel syndrome (IBS) A digestive disease triggered by sensitivities to some foods, among other things. There are two types of IBS. IBS-C has the primary symptom of constipation, and IBS-D has the primary symptom of diarrhea.

Lactose intolerance Inborn defect in digestion and metabolism of lactose, the milk sugar found in milk and dairy products.

"Leaky gut" hypothesis This theory speculates increased intestinal permeability, caused by poor diet choices, inflammatory bowel diseases, antibiotic and chemotherapy drugs, radiation treatments to the abdomen, excess alcohol consumption, non-steroidal anti-inflammatory drugs (NSAIDs), and stress, allows allergens to pass into the bloodstream causing food allergies. This theory is very controversial.

Leukotrienes One type of chemical mediator released during an allergic reaction.

Local Symptoms involving only one specific body system, not all.

Lymphocyte White blood cell in the body which fights allergens, infections, and microorganisms.

Macronutrients An essential substance necessary for growth and health of humans and animals. Examples are carbohydrates, protein, and fats.

Mast cell Type of B cell found in the respiratory tract, intestine, skin, and other body organs and activated in response to foreign invaders during the immune response.

Nonallergic food hypersensitivity Classification defined by the European Academy of Allergology and Clinical Immunology (EAACI) as a food intolerance, food-related medical disorder, or food hypersensitivity.

Oral allergy syndrome Also called pollen-related allergy or a cross-reactivity reaction. Occurs when an individual reacts to the same specific protein allergen found in a food that is also found in other, different sources.

Pathogen Microorganism or substance capable of producing a disease.

Perforate To break down, making a hole through.

Peritonitis Inflammation of the peritoneum, which lines the abdomen.

Phagocyte A cell that has the ability to consume and destroy microorganisms and foreign substances. Phagocytosis is the process of a phagocyte engulfing and destroying a foreign substance.

Prion Disease-causing substance that is not bacterial, fungal, or viral and does not contain any genetic material. A normally harmless protein, a shape change turns it into a rogue protein that entangles other proteins and causes cell damage.

Probiotics A food or substance containing live bacteria that is eaten and helps to restore beneficial bacteria in the gastrointestinal tract. Although probiotics are normally safe to eat, those with a weak immune system or underlying diseases may develop severe infections from the live bacteria. Other side effects include unhealthy metabolic activity, excess stimulation of the immune system, or transfer of genetic information into cells.

Prostaglandins Compounds derived from fatty acids and found in cell membranes. They exhibit a hormone-like effect and are involved in dilation of blood vessels, blood pressure regulation, inflammation, and permeability to fluid and proteins. They also stimulate smooth muscle in the gastrointestinal system and uterus to contract.

Pseudofood allergy syndrome Medical disorder that usually affects adults who diagnose themselves, or were misdiagnosed, and are convinced their symptoms are a food allergy.

RAST (radioallergosorbent test) One of the most accurate tests used for food allergy diagnosis. Drops of blood are placed onto a disk with specific food proteins. The disk is then measured for levels of antibodies that the blood produces. As a rule, the higher the score, the more likely there is a possible allergy to that specific food protein. However, between 50 and 60 percent of positive RAST scores are actually false positives, and 10–30 percent of children with a negative RAST have a food allergy.

Scombroid poisoning The amino acid histidine is present in the gastrointestinal tract of scombroid fish. Scombroid fish include anchovies, bonito, butterfly kingfish, herring, kahawai, mackerel, marlin, pilchards, salmon, sardines, swordfish, and tuna and are the most frequent reason for scrombroid poisoning when they are improperly handled and stored. After these fish are caught, bacteria in the intestine begin to convert histidine into histamine. This conversion happens quickly if the fish is not properly gutted or chilled. Freezing or cooking does not kill this toxin. Symptoms of histamine poisoning usually occur within thirty minutes to a few hours after eating contaminated fish and include a tingling or peppery sensation in the mouth, burning or itching of the skin, diarrhea, faintness, headache, nausea, a rash on the upper body, and vomiting.

Serum IgE concentration Allergy test that measures total IgE level in the blood. Elevated amounts indicate an allergy.

Systemic Affecting the entire body.

Toxin Poisonous substance capable of inducing antibody production.

Ulcerative colitis Inflammatory bowel disease (IBD) that affects the large intestine. Difficult to diagnose and sometimes confused with food allergy or hypersensitivity.

Urticaria See hives.

Vaccine Suspension of microorganisms given for the purpose of stimulating an immune response to develop resistance to an infectious disease. The suspension contains either attenuated or dead microorganisms, a toxin, or extractions from an infectious microorganism.

Vaccination Inoculation with a vaccine to establish resistance to a specific infectious disease.

Variolation Inoculation method used to build immunity against smallpox.

Bibliography

BOOKS

Cruse, Julius M., Robert Lewis. *Atlas of Immunology*. Boca Raton, Florida: CRC Press LLC. 1999.

Gell, P. G. H., and R. R. A. Coombs. *Clinical Aspects of Immunology*, 2nd ed. Oxford: Blackwell, 1968.

Koerner, Celide Barnes, Anne Muñoz-Furlong, and the American Dietetic Association. *Food Allergies*. Minnesota: Chronimed Publishing, 1998.

Melina, Vesanto, Jo Stepaniak, and Dina Aronson. *Food Allergy Survival Guide*. Tennessee: Healthy Living Publications, 2004.

Sicherer, Scott H. *Understanding and Managing Your Child's Food Allergies*. Baltimore, Maryland: The John Hopkins University Press, 2006.

Walsh, William E. *Food Allergies: The Complete Guide to Understanding and Relieving Your Food Allergies*. New York: John Wiley & Sons, Inc., 2000.

Wood, Robert A. *Food Allergies for Dummies*. Indiana: Wiley Publishing, Inc., 2007.

ARTICLES

American Academy of Allergy, Asthma & Immunology. "Food Allergy Statistics" (May 2008). American Academy of Allergy, Asthma, & Immunology web site. http://www.aaaai.org.

Arnold, D. M., M. A. Blajchman, J. DiTomasso, and M. Kulczycki, et al. "Passive Transfer of Peanut Hypersensitivity by Fresh Frozen Plasma." *Archives of Internal Medicine*. 167 (2007): 853–4.

Barrett, J., and P. Gibson. "Clinical Ramifications of Malabsorption of Fructose and Other Short-chain Carbohydrates." *Practical Gastroenterology*. XXXI (2007): 51–65.

Broussard, M. "Everyone's Gone Nuts: The Exaggerated Threat of Food Allergies." *Harper's Magazine,* January 2008. Annotation: 64-65.

Buhner, S., I. Reese, F. Kuehl, H. Lochs, and T. Zuberbier. "Pseudoallergic Reactions in Chronic Urticaria Are Associated with Altered Gastroduodenal Permeability." *Allergy* 59 (2004): 1118–23.

Camargo, C. A., Clark S., Kaplan M. A., et al. "Regional Differences in EpiPen Prescriptions in the United States: The Potential Role of Vitamin D." *The Journal Allergy Clinical Immunology,* 120 (2007): 131–6.

Cox, L. "Felony 'Peanut' Charge Sparks Debate." *ABCNews Internet Ventures* (August 2008), http://abcnews.go.com/Health/AllergiesNews/story?id=4697036>.

DeLano, F., and G. Schmid-Schonbein. "New Molecular Trigger Described for Hypertension, Diabetes." *Hypertension* (September 2008), http://ww.nlm.nih.gov/medlineplus/news/fullstory_66400.

Enrique, E., F. Pineda, T. Malek, et al. "Sublingual Immunotherapy for Hazelnut Food Allergy: A Randomized, Double-Blind, Placebo-Controlled Study with a Standardized Hazelnut Extract." *The Journal of Allergy Clinical Immunology* 116 (2005): 1073–9.

The Food Allergy & Anaphylaxis Network. "Food Allergy Facts and Statistics" (May 2008). The Food Allergy & Anaphylaxis Network, http://www. foodallergy.org.

Food and Agriculture Organization of the United Nations and the World Health Organization. 2000. "Safety Aspects of Genetically Modified Foods of Plant Origin." *Report of a Joint FAO/WHO Expert Consultation on Foods Derived from Biotechnology,* 20–23.

Gary, R., "Peanut and Other Food Allergies—Who Should Be Responsible?" (September 2008). *JAMA Rants, Raves, Reviews* 16:43, http://www.geekzone.co.nz/Jama/2782.

Greer, F. R., S. H. Sicherer, A. W. Burks, et al. "Effects of Early Nutritional Interventions of Atopic Disease in Infants and Children: The Role of Maternal Dietary Restriction, Breastfeeding, Timing of Introduction of Complementary Foods, and Hydrolyzed Formulas." *Pediatrics* 121 (2008): 183–91.

Hallett, R., L. A. D. Haapanen, and S. S. Teuber. "Food Allergies and Kissing." *New England Journal of Medicine* 346 (2002): 1833–4.

Johnston, Martin. "Allergy Blamed For Death at Dinner" (April 2007), http://www.nzherald.co.nz.

Kattan, J. D., K. D. Srivastava, and Z. M. Zou. "Pharmacological and Immunological Effects of Individual Herbs in the Food Allergy Herbal Formula-2 (FAHF-2) on Peanut Allergy." *Phytotherapy Research* 22 (2008): 651–9.

Klement, E., J. Lysy, M. Hoshen, M. Avitan, E. Goldin, and E. Israeli. "Childhood Hygiene Is Associated with the Risk for Inflammatory Bowel Disease: A Population-Based Study." *The American Journal of Gastroenterology* 103 (2008): 1775–82.

Laino, C. "Kissing and Peanut Allergy Dangerous." *WebMD.com* (September 2008), http://www.webmd.com/allergies/news/20060306/kissing-peanut-allergy-dangerous.

Leung, D. Y. M., H. A. Sampson, J. W. Yunginger, et al. "Effect of Anti-IgE Therapy in Patients with Peanut Allergy." *The New England Journal of Medicine* 348 (2003): 986–93.

Madsen, Charlotte. "Prevalence of Food Allergy: An Overview." *Proceedings of the Nutrition Society* 64(2005): 413–417.

Milner, J. D., D. M. Stein, R. McCarter, and R. Y. Moon. "Early Infant Multivitamin Supplementation Is Associated With Increased Risk for Food Allergy and Asthma." *Pediatrics* 114 (2004): 27–32.

National Digestive Diseases Information Clearinghouse. "Facts and Fallacies About Digestive Diseases" (August 2008), http://digestive.niddk.nih.gov/ddiseases/pubs/facts/#ibd.

Nelson, H. S., J. Lahr, R. Rule, A. Bock, and D. Leung. "Treatment of Anaphylactic Sensitivity to Peanuts by Immunotherapy with Injections of Aqueous Peanut Extract." *Journal Allergy Clinical Immunology* 99 (1007): 744–51.

NIH and NIAID. March 13-14, 2006. "Report of the NIH Expert Panel on Food Allergy Research" (September 2008), http://www3.niaid.nih.gov/topics/food Allergy/research/ReportFoodAllergy.

Pearson, D. J. "Pseudo Food Allergy." *British Medical Journal* 292 (1986): 221–2.

Perry, T., M. Conover-Walker, A. Pomés, M. Chapman, and R. Wood. "Distribution of Peanut Allergen in the Environment." *The Journal of Allergy and Clinical Immunology* 113 (2004): 973–6.

Phan, Tri Giang, Simone I. Strasser, and David Koorey, et al. "Passive Transfer of Nut Allergy after Liver Transplantation." *Archives Internal Medicine* 163 (2003): 237–9.

Qin, X. "What Caused the Increase of Autoimmune and Allergic Diseases: A Decreased or an Increased Exposure to Luminal Microbial Components?" *World Journal of Gastroenterology* 13(2008): 1306–7.

Savage, J. H., E. C. Matsui, J. M. Skripak, and R. A. Wood. "The Natural History of Egg Allergy." *The Journal of Allergy and Clinical Immunology* 120 (2007): 1413–7.

Schubert, Charlotte. "Intestinal Worms Show Their Up Side." *Nature News* (September 2008), http://www.nature.com/news/2005/051107/full/news051107-1.

Sicherer, S. H, T. J. Furlong, H. H. Maes, R. J. Desnick, H. A. Samspon, and B. D. Gelb. "Genetics of Peanut Allergy: A Twin Study." *The Journal of Allergy and Clinical Immunology* 106 (2000): 53–6.

Sicherer, Scott H., A. Muñoz-Furlong, R. Murphy, R. Wood, and H. A. Sampson. "Symposium: Pediatric Food Allergy." *Pediatrics* 111 (2003): 1591–4.

Skripak, J. M., E. C. Matsui, K. Mudd, and R. A. Wood. "The Natural History of IgE-Mediated Cow's Milk Allergy". *The Journal of Allergy and Clinical Immunology* 120 (2007): 1172–7.

Stark L. and K. Barrett. "Allergic to Lunchtime." *ABCNews Internet Ventures* (August 2008), http:////abcnews.go.com/Health/AllergiesNews/story?id=4856211.

University of Michigan Health System. "Students with Food Allergies Often Not Prepared." *ScienceDaily* (August 2008), http://www.sciencedaily.com/releases/2008/08/080806081451.

U.S. Food and Drug Administration. "Evidence-based Review System for the Scientific Evaluation of Health Claims" (September 2008). CFSAN/Office of Nutrition, Labeling and Dietary Supplements, http://www.cfsan.fda.gov/~dms/hclmgui5.

U.S. Food and Drug Administration. "Food Allergen Labeling and Consumer Protection Act of 2004" (September 2008), http://www.cfsan.fda.gov/~dms/alrgact.

Vega, C. P. "How Much Gluten Is Too Much? A Best Evidence Review of Celiac Disease." *Medscape Today* (September 2008), http://www.medscape.com/viewarticle/580381.

Willers, S.M., A. H. Wijga, and B. Brunekreef. "Maternal Food Consumption during Pregnancy and the Longitudinal Development of Childhood Asthma." *American Journal of Respiratory and Critical Care Medicine* 131 (2008): 124–31.

Wilson, M. S., M. D. Taylor, and A. Balic, et al. "Suppression of Allergic Airway Inflammation by Helminth-Induced Regulatory T Cells." *Journal of Experimental Medicine* 202 (2005): 1199–212.

Index

About the Author

ALICE C. RICHER, R.D., M.B.A., L.D. is a registered and licensed dietitian who graduated from the University of Rhode Island, trained at Beth Israel Hospital in Boston, MA, and completed her master's degree at Boston College. She currently has a private practice at Spaulding Rehabilitation—Framingham and Braintree outpatient centers, is a medical writer, and is the team dietitian for the MLS soccer team, the New England Revolution. Richer has written numerous articles, conducted professional education courses, appeared on the Norwood cable television parent lecture series, and has been a requested speaker for the Massachusetts Dietetic Association and the Massachusetts Consultant Dietitians. Her award-winning book, *Understanding the Antioxidant Controversy*, with co-author Dr. Paul Milbury, was published in 2007. She is a member of the American Dietetic Association, Massachusetts Dietetic Association, and the American Medical Writers Association.